Lecture Notes on Paediatrics

We dedicate this fourth edition to
Professor Donald Court
whose wisdom and leadership
have contributed so greatly to
child health

Lecture Notes on Paediatrics

S. R. Meadow
MA, BM, FRCP, DCH, DRCOG
Professor of Paediatrics and
Child Health (St James's),
University of Leeds;
Honorary Consultant Paediatrician,
Leeds Area Health Authority (Teaching)

R. W. Smithells
MB, FRCP, FRCP(E), DCH
Professor of Paediatrics and
Child Health (Leeds General Infirmary),
University of Leeds;
Honorary Consultant Paediatrician,
Leeds Area Health Authority (Teaching)

Fourth edition

Blackwell Scientific Publications
OXFORD LONDON
EDINBURGH BOSTON MELBOURNE

© 1973, 1975, 1978, 1981
Blackwell Scientific Publications
Editorial offices:
Osney Mead, Oxford, OX2 0EL
8 John Street, London, WC1N 2ES
9 Forrest Road, Edinburgh, EH1 2QH
52 Beacon Street, Boston
  Massachusetts 02108, USA
99 Barry Street, Carlton
  Victoria 3053, Australia

First published 1973
Revised reprint 1974
Second edition 1975
Reprinted 1977
Third edition 1978
Reprinted 1981
Fourth edition 1981

Portuguese translation 1980

Printed in Great Britain at
The Alden Press, Oxford
and bound at
Kemp Hall Bindery, Oxford

DISTRIBUTORS

USA
  Blackwell Mosby Book Distributors
  11830 Westline Industrial Drive
  St Louis, Missouri 63141

Canada
  Blackwell Mosby Book Distributors
  120 Melford Drive, Scarborough
  Ontario, M1B 2X4

Australia
  Blackwell Scientific Book Distributors
  214 Berkley Street, Carlton
  Victoria 3053

British Library
Cataloguing in Publication Data

British Library Cataloguing in
Publication Data
_____

Meadow, Roy
  Lecture notes on paediatrics—4th ed.
  1. Pediatrics
  I. Title II. Smithells, R.W.
  618.92   RJ45

ISBN 0–632–00824–5

Contents

Preface to Fourth Edition

In preparing this fourth edition of Lecture Notes the book has been extensively revised and updated, new illustrations have been added and several chapters completely rewritten. By removing dead wood we have been able to allow greater exposure for new and more important branches of paediatrics without significant increase in size. We have been determined to keep the book small enough to fit into the pocket of a white coat (or a jacket, if white coats become unfashionable). We are pleased to know that over 50,000 pockets have accommodated it so far.

Leeds
1981

Roy Meadow
Dick Smithells

Preface to First Edition

Paediatrics concerns the health and illness of children. Children make up more than one-fifth of our population and an even higher proportion of a general practitioner's working day. It is often in childhood that the patterns of adult health and disease have their origins. Paediatrics rubs shoulders with education and with the social services. It is concerned with children and their families first, and with disease second.

Medical education is a continuing process which starts at school and should not end before retirement. The pre-registration year ensures that the new medical student is not 'let loose upon the public'. Today's medical students should therefore be expected to absorb less factual material than did their ancestors. This is a small book, intended to live in the pocket of a white coat rather than on a bookshelf. It describes the pattern of childhood growth and development and conditions which are either common, important or interesting. This factual framework is set against the changing pattern of paediatric practice, the services available for children and the needs of society.

Our aim has been to provide a framework of paediatric knowledge sufficient for the medical student during the paediatric appointment; but it must be grafted on to preliminary experience of adult medicine and surgery. We have deliberately placed more emphasis on diagnosis than on treatment; therapeutic details are best learned by caring for sick children.

For medical students who use this book, far more important than further reading is the need to spend time and trouble getting to know children, and developing the techniques of examining children and talking to them and their parents. This applies also to the many other groups who work with children—therapists, nurses and health visitors—for whom we hope this book will provide a useful supplement to their lectures and their work.

Acknowledgments

We thank our colleagues for their advice and help, and in particular   Dr C C Bailey,   Mr J M Beck,   Dr J M H Buckler, Mrs L M Levett, Dr J M Littlewood, Mr F D McAuley and Dr S H Roussounis.

The figures were drawn by Mr H Grayshon Lumby, MSIA, and most of the photographs were prepared by the Department of Medical Photography at the University of Leeds, and St James's University Hospital.

We are grateful to a number of colleagues who have helped with illustrations, particularly Mrs G Levell, Dr J M Littlewood, Professor V Dubowitz and Professor J M Tanner.

We are indebted to our assistant Mrs Wendy Pearson, whose efficiency, thoughtfulness and stamina have ensured that the manuscript has been completed in time.

Chapter 1

The Child as a Patient

HISTORY TAKING

The child's history covers the same ground as that of an adult patient, with some important additions. The start is similar. We need to know the **name, age and sex** of the patient and the main reason for the consultation, i.e. the **main complaint**. Find out and write on the notes what the child is called at home, e.g. 'Larry'. This avoids anyone greeting him with an unfamiliar formal name—'Good morning, Lawrence'. Similarly, it is courteous to refer to the mother as 'Mrs Jackson'—not 'Mother' or 'Mum'.

The interview will be more productive if the parent and child are sitting comfortably and at ease; a young child is likely to feel more secure on a parental knee. Communication is best if the doctor and parent sit at right angles to each other rather than in a 'headmaster–pupil' confrontation.

The **history of the present condition** (including a review of the systems) will usually be obtained from the parent, though any child who can talk may be able to contribute additional useful information. A 5-year-old may agree to 'put your hand where it hurts'. Older children should be seen on their own for a few minutes with the parent out of the room. This allows direct doctor–child communication, increases the child's self-confidence and ensures better cooperation with future management. It also enables the doctor to speak to the parent alone without the child feeling slighted: 'Please will you wait outside while I talk with your mummy, and then she'll wait outside while I talk with you.'

It is usually best to listen to the story of the presenting condition before asking about the family and perinatal history, because the presenting condition is what the parent wants to talk about first. A detailed account of the symptoms is the vital part of any history, and it is important to find out how the problems affect the child's life. School is the equivalent of an adult's employment. School attendance and progress are important variables, and the name of the school should be noted so that a report from the school teacher can be obtained or a letter written to the school doctor if necessary.

Ask for the parent's own ideas about what is the matter with the child. Sometimes it will enable you to assuage an unnecessary anxiety; at other times it may lead to a correct diagnosis you had not considered. Mothers are more likely than anyone else to understand their babies' cries, and research shows that babies can 'talk'. They have a different cry for hunger, for pain, etc.; and the characteristic cries of meningitis, Down's syndrome and hypothyroidism are all different. The mother will usually know when the cry is abnormal and sometimes will be able to suggest a reason.

It is often helpful, especially if psychological problems are suspected, to ask 'What kind of boy (girl) is he (she)?' The answer may be 'a worrier', 'placid', 'never still', 'obsessional'. If you then ask 'Who does he take after?', it often provides useful insight for the parent. It is also helpful to know what the child does in his spare time and whether he is by nature gregarious or solitary.

Previous medical history should include not only details of bad illnesses, operations or hospital attendances, but also any allergies or drug sensitivities. It is worth remembering that a history of rubella is extremely unreliable: many other minor infections simulate rubella. The immunisation history must be included; it may help to exclude a suspected condition, and it identifies those families in need of advice about further immunisation. Triple vaccine is often referred to as '3-in-1'. BCG and smallpox vaccination scars can be recognised on inspection.

Family history should include:

1   The number and ages of the siblings and parents.

2   Whether any other member of the family has or has had the same condition as the child, whether it be a rash and fever (? has the child caught the same infection), or

six digits on each hand (? has the child an inherited condition which runs in the family).

3   What illnesses the parents and close relatives have had, in order to allay needless worries. The parents may worry that their child's stomach ache is caused by stomach cancer, because grandma recently died with it.

4   The presence or absence of consanguinity, because rare inherited conditions are more likely if the parents are related.

The **perinatal history** should provide details of the prenancy and first week of life. In the pregnancy, establish its length (normal is 40 weeks) and any maternal infections, illnesses, or abnormalities. Details of the delivery should include the place of birth, presentation (head or breech), type (spontaneous, forceps or caesarean section) and the birth weight. Any abnormality of the neonatal period is soon discovered by asking if the baby needed special care (in an incubator, or a special care unit) after birth. A healthy baby would have been allowed to be with his mother for the first day, and be allowed home with his mother at the planned time. Slowness to feed in the early days and cyanotic or apnoeic attacks are sometimes indicators of brain damage.

The **developmental history** is almost unique to paediatrics. It is important, particularly for young or handicapped children. It includes details of the times at which skills such as walking and talking were acquired (full details in Chapter 5).

The **social history** is obtained, after establishing rapport with the parents, by talking with them about their life, their home, their work and their problems. Find out the father's job (it is a useful financial guide), and find out exactly what the job entails: a 'lorry driver' may be a local parcel deliverer or a long-distance lorry driver who is away from home much of the time. Does the mother work and, if she does, who looks after the child? If the mother is now a housewife, what was her job before she married? If she was a nurse, she will have a different level of knowledge and a different need for information. Three particular areas must be explored which have a direct influence on the child's development:

1   The family composition: are the mother and father

living together, or is this a single-parent family who in our society are 'the poorest of the poor'.

2   The financial situation: is the family financially viable, with a regular income, or are they dependent on grants from the social services department.

3   Housing: have they a home of their own, and if so, what sort; or are they living with relatives or in a hostel? Satisfactory housing should have not more than 1·5 persons per room, a supply of hot water and indoor sanitation.

We each find some parents easy to interview, and others difficult. It is as well to get into the habit of blaming oneself if the history is unclear. If you are tempted to label someone a 'bad historian', remember that a historian is the person who collects and records the history!

IMMIGRANT FAMILIES

For many centuries new immigrant communities have formed an important part of Britain's population. The main medical problems and misunderstandings occur in relation to the large groups from the Indian subcontinent whose language and culture are poorly understood by people in Britain.

In general, particular sects of immigrants tend to live together, so that certain towns and cities may have a preponderance of one or other sect (e.g. Gujarati Indians in Leicester and Pakistanis in Bradford). It is worth finding out if local immigrants are mainly of a particular sect or religion and to be aware of some of the differences. The main Asian groups are from:

(a) North-east Pakistan and Bangladesh, usually Muslim (Islam religion)

(b) Gujarat in north-west India, mainly Hindu

(c) Punjab in northern India, usually Sikh.

There are several important medical aspects:

1   *Names*

Selecting the appropriate and polite name can be difficult. Sikh boys have the complementary name Singh, and girls Kaur. The personal name precedes the complementary name and the subcaste name (surname) follows it, e.g. Davindar Kaur Bhumbra. The Hindu naming system is somewhat similar. Devi for girls, and Lal for boys, are common complementary names, and may be joined on to the first personal name e.g. Arima Devi Chopra becomes Arimadevi Chopra. Some Sikhs and Hindus will not use a subcaste name. Muslim names are more difficult; often there is no shared family name. Males have a religious title (e.g. Mohammed or Abdul) which may precede or follow the personal name. Females have a title (e.g. Begum or Bibi) and a personal name. It is discourteous to use the religious name or title on its own; it must be coupled with the personal name. (In close friendship the personal name is used on its own without the religious name or title.)

2 Contact with foreign diseases

Most children will have been born and brought up in Britain. But if the child has recently arrived in the country, or returned from visiting relatives in the parents' homeland, he is at risk for unusual illnesses (malaria is seen in children returning from Pakistan and hookworm in those from tropical and subtropical regions) and for diseases which are more common abroad (e.g. tuberculosis in India and Pakistan).

3 Racial susceptibility to disease

Some diseases are exclusive to certain races, e.g. sickle-cell disease in negroes. More commonly a disease is simply more likely in particular races, e.g. thalassaemia major which is common in Pakistanis, and very common in Cypriots. Consanguinity (marrying a blood relative) is common in some cultures, particularly Muslims. The offspring have an increased chance of receiving the same recessive gene from each parent, and of developing an otherwise rare genetically determined disease.

4 Food

Asian families are prone to nutritional problems because of the difficult compromise they have to achieve between their religious beliefs and the British food industry. Orthodox Hindus are vegetarian, less strict Hindus avoid beef, and any food which has been processed with utensils that may have been in contact with beef. Muslims avoid pork with similar strictness, and any meat must be killed in a special way (Halal). Muslim children at puberty may join the Ramazan month-long fast each year. Although Asians are considerable users of butter, they will not use margarine (which is a notable source of vitamin D for many British families).

5 *Customs*

Asian women avoid exposure to sunlight; vitamin D deficiency is common in pregnancy and is a risk for their newborn babies. As the girls reach puberty they adopt traditional clothes which shield their limbs and skin from sunlight; the chance of rickets is increased. Orthodox Muslim women are relatively confined to the home, and lead a restricted life; very often the husband will be responsible for all outside activities including taking the child to a doctor or hospital. The person accompanying the child to the clinic may be the most senior male member of the family or the best at speaking English, yet know little of the child's problem or the mother's worries.

Enquiring about the racial background or the family cultural and religious beliefs should not be a source of embarrassment; nor is it a basis for unfair discrimination. In practice we behave as if all children are born equal— then we respect and cater for their differences and difficulties. We want an aristocracy of achievement.

EXAMINATION

The rigid rules that have been learnt for examining adults have to be bent when applied to small babies, frightened toddlers and nervous children. The young child has to be charmed and seduced before he will allow a useful examination. A baby responds to comforting noises and smiles, an older child to gentle friendly talk and play.

Avoid separating the mother and child, and avoid asking young children to lie down on an examination couch. If it is necessary, wait until the child is less fearful towards the end of the examination.

Examination of the school child is not difficult. Most are cooperative and confident provided a parent is there. Those over the age of 10 may prefer more privacy, but although they may prefer to be examined without their parent watching, they are usually comforted by their presence nearby.

Pre-school children are more difficult. The doctor must be an opportunist, adapting his examination to the openings that present. The infant should be examined as he allows; if he is quiet listen to the heart, if his eyes are open look at his eyes. It is often best to touch and examine first a young child's hands, for they are used to that, before attempting to examine the child fully. It is unwise to demand at the start 'remove all the clothes' if this is going to result in prolonged crying—small children don't like taking their clothes off. More information is obtained from a partly clothed contented child sitting on his mother's knee, than from a screaming naked child on an examination couch.

Children worry about any instruments so these need to be explained and a running commentary kept up for the benefit of child and parent. The grim-faced silent doctor spells doom, whilst the calm friendly one radiates optimistic confidence with his 'Your hair is nice', 'Your heart is strong', 'Your blood pressure is very healthy'. Gaiety may be out of place when a child is ill but it is better to be buoyant and cheerful than unresponsive and dull. Compliments for good teeth, a good figure and well-cared-for hands and feet are good reinforcing health education.

The techniques for examining the different systems are given in the chapters about those systems. All new patients should have their height and weight measured and checked against the normal range for their age. Poor growth or low weight relative to height may be a sign of serious illness. Note is taken of the child's cleanliness and clothes, and of evidence of scalp infestation or bitten nails that may be signs of other problems. Routine urine examination by Dipstix and microscopy (p. 213) is obligatory. The temperature is usually taken rectally during the first year of life, in the axilla up to the age of 5 and orally in school children.

CHILDREN IN HOSPITAL

The hazards of illness are obvious to everyone; the hazards of hospitalisation and of parent–child separation are less obvious, yet sometimes as serious. The pre-school child, particularly from 1 to $3\frac{1}{2}$ years, needs his mother. She is needed to make the world around intelligible to him, and to act as a barrier to environmental stress, ensuring it comes gradually. When separated from her he is old enough to grieve over his loss, yet neither old enough to understand the reason nor to be comforted by others. The young child admitted to hospital may go through three stages (Fig. 1):

1 Protest, on the first day, as he cries for his mother and shouts for her return, perhaps standing up in the cot shaking the rails angrily.

2 Withdrawal, as he curls up in his cot quietly mourning over his loss. He refuses to eat or play with others, but may get some comfort from a dummy or favourite cuddly bit of material. The mourning phase can last for many days.

3 Denial—of the memory of his mother. He is superficially happy, making quick casual friendships with anyone, holding hands with and kissing the doctors and nurses. By this stage the mother–child relationship has been damaged, and when the child goes home a new bond will have to be fashioned. Meanwhile, there may be tantrums, nightmares, food refusal, bed wetting and other behaviour problems.

Prolonged separation may produce prolonged harm including physical and emotional illness in later life, delinquency and unstable marriages. Therefore management of the ill child, particularly those pre-school children who are most vulnerable to mother–child separation, involves:

1 Avoiding hospital admission unless it is essential.

2 Reducing the length of any admission to a minimum. The child is sent home still ill if there is no need for special hospital investigation or care. Many operations such as herniotomy and orchidopexy and procedures such as jejunal biopsy are done as 'day cases', the child being admitted, operated upon and sent home within 9 hours so that overnight stay is not needed.

Protest   Withdrawal   Denial

Fig. 1. A young child's response to separation from his mother. He eventually denies the presence of his mother and superficially appears happy.

3 Encouraging parents to visit their ill child in hospital at any time (unrestricted visiting), and creating facilities for mothers to sleep in hospital with their child.

The long-term damage from mother–child separation may have been over-emphasised. We now realise that the factors leading to separation during the early critical years of development often persist and so continue to disrupt the child's life (e.g. continued parental problems and marital difficulties). Moreover, there is no doubt that the risks of repeated hospital admissions are greater for those from disadvantaged backgrounds. It is not always possible to identify the factor most responsible for affecting a child's development. However, for many children hospital admission is a contributory factor.

Because of the risk of being upset by an unpleasant and sudden separation, parents should be encouraged to ensure that their children experience early in life a brief and *happy* separation, perhaps with a grandparent or other relative. In that way the child may come to realise that temporary separation from the mother need not be disastrous.

For those children who have to be in hospital there is much that can be done to reduce the stress. Children are grouped together so that they may be looked after by qualified staff specially trained in the care of children. Teachers and play leaders are used to organize education and play. The segregation from adults allows the children's wards to be made more homely. Good children's wards give an impression more of happy chaos than of highly organized medical technology (which is in fact going on).

MANAGEMENT

The child

An important part of the doctor's role is to anticipate and prevent needless pain or anxiety for the child. All children dislike 'pricks' whether they be venepunctures or intramuscular injections. Some are necessary but they must be kept to a minimum. Children respect and require honesty. It is wrong to say that painful procedures don't hurt; the child later feels tricked and trust is lost.

Fig. 2. Hospital can be like home.

Nevertheless, suggestion plays a part in most things so it is fair to minimize the pain—'it will hurt a little, just at the beginning, but not a lot'. Strange apparatus should be kept out of sight until it is used, then it must be explained, 'the X-ray machine is held up by a very strong metal rope which cannot break—it takes a photograph and does not hurt'. A child who must keep still (for an EEG) may be best on mother's knee. A young child who must keep very still (e.g. for CAT scan) may need an anaesthetic.

The parents

The mother of an ill child tends to be regarded as either 'over-anxious' or 'irresponsible'. The land between in which the parents show what most doctors and nurses consider 'reasonable' concern, is scanty and rarely inhabited. Anxiety is normal; excessive anxiety and aggression often stem from lack of information. The doctor dealing with anxious parents needs compassion, tact and skill to help them.

Parental guilt at the time of a child's illness is common—they may have brought a weak congenitally handicapped child into the world, there may have been an accident involving the child for which they feel negligent, or an illness which they think would not have happened if they had 'given more vitamins', or 'kept her out of the rain'. These worries need to be ventilated and the doctor's role is that of listener and helper. The guilt feelings and the widespread feeling of inferiority to doctors and nurses make communication difficult, so the doctor must actively encourage them to talk, and anticipate their problems.

Because the general level of the parents' medical information may be 30 years out of date, their worries may be unsuspected by sophisticated medical and nursing staff. They may think that vomiting means something wrong with the abdomen, not knowing that it is a common feature of most febrile illnesses of childhood. They will worry if their child is not eating, almost as if he will perish from starvation, and therefore they need to be told that an ill child can manage well on drinks alone for a few days. It is worth remembering that the press and television tend to create topical diseases, and that parents may be worrying about rare conditions such as autism or leukaemia because of recent publicity.

Parents worry needlessly about rare diseases because they see tests done which are neither explained nor reported to them. They fear leukaemia because a blood test has been done. The level of explanation varies with each family. The language must be relevant to that family, and like all important messages must be repeated on another occasion. Many parents may want to know the name of the child's illness, but all parents want to know how it will affect the child. Similarly they are more concerned about what the surgeon *did* than what the child *had*. The days of the omniscient doctor are on the decline. Most parents want a kind and conscientious human being to help their child rather than a mystical god.

It is honest and respectable to admit: 'I don't know what the matter is' provided that one goes on to say 'but I do know what we must do to find out and to help.'

Episodes of illness should leave the parents more confident in themselves and in the Health Service, not less. Doctors and nurses must avoid taking over the child and leaving the parents without a role and without self respect. Often the parents make the major contribution to management e.g. insulin administration and diet for a young diabetic, or postural drainage and physiotherapy for a child with cystic fibrosis. And for the diffident and not so confident there are always things a parent can do, and will do better than us, and we should say so. 'Please will you put on his nappy, you'll do it better than me.' However poor the mother is at mothering there will always be something we can find to praise in her care. This we must do—she is the only mother that child will ever have, and she is the best that the child will ever have. In our dealings with her we must make sure she emerges proud, confident, and competent with her child.

Further reading

Apley J., Mac Keith R. C. & Meadow S. R. *The Child and His Symptoms,* Chapters 21–24. Blackwell Scientific Publications.

Henley A. *Asian Patients in Hospital and at Home.* Kings Fund Publishing Office, London.

Various explanatory publications about immigrants are published by the Community Relations Commission, 15/16 Bedford Street, London WC2E 9HX.

Chapter 2

The Newborn Baby

The first 24 hours of life present greater opportunities to save life and prevent handicap than any other time between birth and death. It is therefore essential that all doctors should be capable of making a competent examination of newborn babies, of recognising ill health and congenital defect at the earliest possible moment and of dealing with those problems which demand immediate action. The **examination of the infant at birth** is usually carried out by the midwife to determine (a) that there is nothing to interfere with the establishment of normal respiration, and (b) that there are no gross external deformities. If there is any evidence of ill health, prompt examination by a doctor is necessary. At no other time of life does illness, or suspicion of illness, demand such urgent attention. Minor delays may have major consequences. This is why all very small or sick babies in a maternity unit are gathered together in a special-care baby unit, where experienced medical and nursing staff and specialised equipment are available round the clock. Complex problems may require transfer to more specialised regional neonatal intensive care units.

Within the first 24–48 hours of life every baby should be examined in detail by a doctor. This **routine examination** is a screening procedure intended to assess general health and to recognise congenital defects promptly. The examination will be most satisfactory if it is carried out when the baby is awake but contented, a happy frame of mind most likely to be encountered shortly after a feed. His general health can best be judged without disturbing him by observing his colour, the posture in which he lies, the way he moves and (if he cries) by the nature of his cry. Examination of muscle tone is also informative, but can often be inferred from observations of posture and move-

Fig. 3. Neonatal intensive care.

ment. The normal colour, posture and cry cannot be described: they can be learned from newborn babies.

Some important observations made routinely by the midwife will also help the doctor to assess the baby's health. These include measurement of weight, length and head circumference, and observation of urine and meconium, both of which are usually passed within 24 hours of birth. Failure to do so should prompt a search for obstructive lesions, though an infant who has passed meconium before birth may not do so again until 36–48 hours after birth. Meconium changes to milk stools on days 3–4. The umbilical cord has usually separated by 7 days but may take a few days longer.

The routine examination of the newborn should

include attention to the points listed in Table 1. Such examination will reveal most, but not all defects. Congenital heart disease especially may not be detectable for days or weeks. Renal tract anomalies, unless gross, are not detected until urinary infection supervenes and points the need for pyelography. Metabolic disease may need to be sought by biochemical testing, either on a population basis, as in screening for phenylketonuria, or in selected infants if there is a relevant family history.

Table 1. Routine examination of newborn infant

Examination	Conditions sought
Weight and length	Intrauterine malnutrition ('Light for dates')
Head circumference, sutures, fontanelles	Hydrocephalus: microcephaly
Facial features and ears	Malformation syndromes (e.g. Down's): facial palsy
Eyes	Glaucoma: cataract: corneal opacities
Mouth	Cleft palate: congenital teeth
Jaw	Abnormal size or position of mandible
Chest	Abnormalities of lungs
Heart	Congenital heart disease: mediastinal displacement
Abdomen	Abnormal masses (e.g. cystic kidneys)
Perineum	Genital anomalies: anal anomalies
Hips	Instability or dislocation
Femoral pulses	Coarctation of aorta
Back	Spina bifida: dermal sinus: post-anal dimple
Limbs	Talipes: abnormal long bones and digits: palmar creases
Reflexes and responses / Certain physical features	Assessment of gestational age (see p. 28)

CONGENITAL MALFORMATIONS

About 2% of all babies are born with serious congenital defects, sufficient to threaten life, to cause permanent handicap, or to require surgical correction. Malformations therefore form a major cause of perinatal and infant death, and constitute one of the greatest problems in paediatrics (Fig. 4). Defects of the central nervous system and heart account for more than half the total. Most of the common defects are described in the relevant chapters: here some general principles will be considered.

Distressingly little is known of the causes of congenital abnormalities. Single gene defects and chromosome anomalies account for 10–20% of the total. A small number are attributable to intrauterine infections (e.g. cytomegalovirus, rubella), fewer to teratogenic drugs and even fewer to ionising radiation. The causes of most common defects remain unknown, although some aetiological

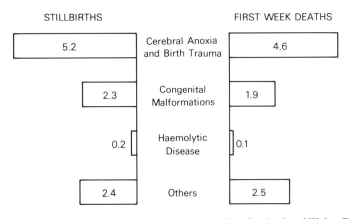

Fig. 4. Causes of perinatal mortality, England and Wales. Rates per 1000 total births.

factors are known. For example, some defects are more common in certain ethnic groups, socio-economic groups, or at some maternal ages and parities than others. It is believed that most non-genetic defects arise from the simultaneous action of many adverse factors upon a susceptible embryo.

The incidence of serious defects and chromosomal anomalies amongst early spontaneous abortuses is very high. Nature has devised a fairly efficient system for terminating at the first possible moment pregnancies which are doomed to failure. It can be shown, for example, that at least 90% of mongols and a much higher proportion of embryos with sex chromosome anomalies are aborted. Live-born, malformed infants therefore represent the small minority for which this mechanism has failed.

Early diagnosis of congenital anomalies is necessary because:
1   it may influence the management of pregnancy and delivery;
2   prompt treatment may be necessary;
3   parents need early information and advice.

Major anomalies can sometimes be diagnosed before birth. The development of polyhydramnios (excess amniotic fluid) will prompt abdominal ultrasound scan or X-ray which may reveal multiple pregnancy or anencephaly (absence of cerebral hemispheres and cranial vault). Oligohydramnios raises the possibility of deficient fetal urinary output, as in renal agenesis. Techniques available for pre-natal diagnosis include X-rays, ultrasound, amniocentesis, amniography and fetoscopy. X-rays show the big head of hydrocephalus and the short limbs of some generalised bone dystrophies. Ultrasound techniques are being refined to reveal ever finer structural detail and can, for example, demonstrate congenital heart disease in utero. Amniocentesis, which can be performed at 14–16 weeks of pregnancy, allows chemical analysis of the fluid (especially for alpha-fetoprotein (AFP) which is increased with neural tube defects), histochemical studies of fixed (fetal) cells, and cell culture leading to fetal karyotyping. Routine testing of *serum* AFP followed by selective amniocentesis may soon make neural tube defects in viable babies very rare. However, prenatal diagnosis of defects is only useful if followed by abortion of abnormal fetuses. It is not preventing malformations but preventing the live birth of malformed babies. Amniography outlines the fetus in utero by injecting radio-opaque material into the amniotic fluid. Fetoscopy, still an experimental technique, permits visualisation of the fetus and the taking of fetal blood samples for diagnosis (e.g. thalassaemia).

After birth, most congenital defects will be revealed by the careful clinical examination already described. Others can only be suspected when they give rise to symptoms such as vomiting, cyanosis, jaundice, or failure to pass urine or meconium. When a congenital defect has been firmly diagnosed, the information has to be given to the parents together with an indication of the prognosis.

The news that a baby is deformed is a great shock to the parents. Even minor anomalies are seen as major tragedies. At the first interview detailed explanations will not be grasped. If the baby is to be transferred to another hospital for early surgery, the mother must have a chance to see her infant before removal. She will need frequent progress reports on the baby until she is able to visit. The closer the contact the parents maintain with the baby, the less likely are they to reject it if there is a residual handicap. If the baby survives, the parents need patient explanation of the care needed and how to recognise any problems that are likely to arise. They will almost certainly feel that the infant's deformity is somehow their fault, and will wonder why it happened to them.

They will need advice about the recurrence risks if they plan another child later on. For easily recognisable conditions in which a genetic (or non-genetic) basis is clearly established, the family doctor or paediatrician can provide this information. For more complex problems reference to a *genetic counselling* clinic is advisable. The three basic essentials for counselling are:

1 a firmly established diagnosis, which is often more difficult than it sounds;
2 a full family history;
3 ample time to elicit facts and anxieties, and to explain recurrence risks, prenatal tests and other relevant issues.

All this implies ready access to doctors and nurses who can listen and answer, and who can at least give the appearance of having unlimited time to spare. Parents of seriously handicapped children can often help one another through membership of parents' associations or organisations. Such associations exist not only for the parents of children with serious malformations such as spina bifida, but also for those with mental handicap, cerebral palsy, muscular dystrophy, cystic fibrosis, leukaemia, infantile autism, deafness, blindness and other disorders.

In summary, whenever a malformed baby is born the parents want to know:

1 exactly what is the matter, in terms they can grasp;

2   what can the doctors do about it;
3   what can the parents do about it;
4   what is the outlook for this child;
5   what is the outlook for any other children that may follow;
6   finally, parents want to know why it happened, but only exceptionally can this be answered.

PERINATAL ASPHYXIA

Before birth the fetus is dependent for his oxygen supply upon (a) a normal oxygen tension in the mother's blood; (b) a healthy placenta firmly attached to the uterine wall; and (c) unobstructed blood flow through the umbilical vessels. After birth, the newborn baby's oxygenation depends upon (a) a functioning respiratory centre; (b) a patent airway; and (c) healthy heart and lungs. Interference with one or more of these functions is likely to lead to hypoxia, either before birth or immediately afterwards (see Fig. 5). Hypoxia before birth is recognised by the signs of fetal distress of which the most important are

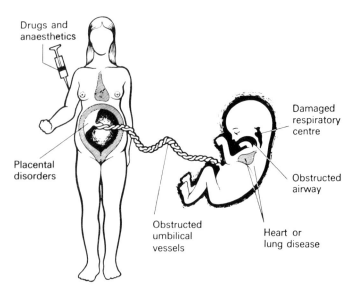

Drugs and anaesthetics

Placental disorders

Obstructed umbilical vessels

Damaged respiratory centre

Obstructed airway

Heart or lung disease

Fig. 5. Causes of birth asphyxia.

bradycardia and meconium staining of the liquor. Continuous monitoring of fetal heart rate in relation to uterine contractions is helpful. More direct evidence of hypoxia and acidosis is now sought by estimations of pO_2 and pH on blood samples obtained from the fetal scalp when the cervix is sufficiently widely dilated. After birth, hypoxia is recognised by alterations of pulse, respiration, colour, tone and reflex irritability, the last being tested either by slapping the feet or inserting a catheter into the nares. It is usual to score these five attributes on a 0, 1, 2 scale, the total score ranging from 0 for a dead baby to 10 for one in the pink of condition. This is the Apgar score, named after the late Dr Virginia Apgar who described the method. Details are shown in Table 2. The score is

Table 2. Apgar score

Sign	0	1	2
Heart rate	Absent	Below 100/min	100/min or higher
Respiratory effort	Nil	Slow, irregular	Regular, with cry
Muscle tone	Limp	Some tone in limbs	Active movements
Reflex irritability	Nil	Grimace only	Cry
Colour	Pallor or generalised cyanosis	Body pink, extremities blue	Pink all over

normally assessed 1 minute after birth, and at 5 and 10 minutes if necessary. A score of 7 or higher is satisfactory and no intervention is called for. A score of 3 or less indicates severe hypoxia and impending death.

It will be seen in Table 3 that hypoxia, by damaging the respiratory centre, may cause further hypoxia. This downhill spiral can only be reversed by improving the oxygen supply to the brain before the circulation stops, the most efficient method being endotracheal intubation and positive pressure insufflation. Apgar scores in the intermediate range of 4–6 usually indicate the need for simple measures, including clearing the airway by suction, gentle stimulation of the baby, and the administration of oxygen by face mask. Naloxone hydrochloride should be given, 0·01 mg/kg i.m., if the mother has been given pethidine or morphine derivatives during labour.

Table 3. Perinatal oxygen supply

Requirements	Potential threats
A. *Before Birth*	
Normal oxygen tension in mother's blood	Advanced heart or lung disease
	Unskilled anaesthesia
Healthy placenta, firmly attached	Placental insufficiency
	Placental abruption ⎱ (premature separation
	Placental praevia ⎰ of the placenta)
Unobstructed umbilical vessels	Prolapsed cord
	Ruptured cord; knotted cord
	Prolonged labour
B. *At birth*	
Functioning respiratory centre	Intracranial haemorrhage
	Cerebral hypoxia
	Respiratory depressant drugs
Patent airway	Mucus, blood, meconium in airway
	Retrognathia (jaw too far back)
	Micrognathia (jaw too small)
	Choanal atresia (blocked nasopharynx)
Healthy heart and lungs	Diaphragmatic hernia
	Major anomalies of the lungs
	Severe congenital heart lesions

The fetus deprived of oxygen responds initially by increased respiratory effort. If this is unavailing, respiration becomes more and more feeble and then stops (primary apnoea). After a short time respiration begins again and continues until the last gasp, which is followed by secondary (terminal) apnoea. In the latter, the Apgar score is likely to be only 1 or 2—the baby is pale, limp and unresponsive with bradycardia.

Newborn babies are capable of utilizing some anaerobic metabolic pathways and can therefore tolerate hypoxia of more severe degree than can older children or adults. Nevertheless, the condition is serious and requires urgent and skilled attention because the brain is the tissue most sensitive to oxygen lack, and severe hypoxia may cause death, mental defect, cerebral palsy or other permanent neurological disorders. The principles of treatment of severe birth asphyxia include the maintenance of normal pO_2 by assisted ventilation and normal pH by i.v. sodium bicarbonate. Intermittent positive pressure ventilation (IPPV) should be instituted in any baby with terminal apnoea or not breathing within 2 minutes of birth. Subsequently arterial pO_2 will need monitoring, with ventilatory assistance by continuous positive airways pressure (CPAP) using a Gregory head box or by a ventilator. The combination of continuous monitoring of pO_2 and pH by cutaneous electrodes or indwelling umbilical arterial catheters and obsessional correction of deviations from normal have vastly improved the prognosis for severely asphyxiated newborns, especially those of low birth weight. Nevertheless, if the institution of adequate ventilation is delayed, the prognosis is less good. Convulsions following birth asphyxia are a bad prognostic sign.

BIRTH INJURY

The term birth injury usually refers to physical injury, as distinct from the chemical injury of hypoxia, hyperbilirubinaemia and hypoglycaemia. The distinction between intracranial birth injury and hypoxia is not clear, since hypoxia can cause capillary damage leading to intraventricular haemorrhage, and the haemorrhage resulting from tears of the falx cerebri or tentorium cerebelli may damage the respiratory centre and lead to hypoxia. Intracranial birth injury may occur if the baby is very small (with soft skull and brain) or very large (with consequent mechanical problems); if labour is very rapid, causing rapid compression and decompression of the head; if there is malpresentation of the fetus; or if there is difficult forceps delivery. These may cause intracerebral, subarachnoid or subdural haemorrhage, leading to death or survival with brain damage. Nothing can be done directly to stop bleeding. Treatment is as for severe hypoxia but is often unavailing.

Fractures

Skull fracture is not uncommon but is usually linear without displacement, causing no symptoms and needing no treatment. A localised, depressed fracture is usually best treated by elevation of the bone, although if there are no focal signs it may heal without sequelae.

Apart from the skull, fractures are only likely to arise when there is difficulty delivering the infant's shoulders, when the bones likely to break are the clavicle and the humerus. These fractures always unite without deformity.

Cephalhaematoma

Cephalhaematoma results from bleeding between a skull bone and the overlying periosteum. One or both parietals are commonly affected, the occipital occasionally, the frontals never. The swelling is soft and fluctuant and conforms in shape and position to a cranial bone (Fig. 6).

Fig. 6. Cephalhaematoma of the right parietal region.

It cannot cross a suture. Some resolve within a few weeks: others calcify, especially around the periphery, and take longer to go. In neither case is any treatment required, beyond explanation and reassurance to the parents.

Subaponeurotic haemorrhage

24   This disorder is rare but serious. It may occur in babies

with blood clotting defects (e.g. factor V deficiency). The bleeding occurs into the 'scalping' layer and spreads over the whole surface of the vault of the skull. As the newborn's total blood volume is about 300 ml, he can easily bleed to death into the subaponeurotic layer. Rapid recognition, prompt transfusion, and the correction of any clotting defect will save lives.

Nerve palsies

The same shoulder-stretching force may injure the brachial plexus and cause nerve palsies. The more common Erb's palsy results from stretching of the upper roots of the plexus. The arm lies straight and limp beside the body, internally rotated and with the fingers flexed (usually referred to as the waiter's tip, or in shadier parts the policeman's tip, position, but probably only seen in these gentlemen if they have brachial plexus lesions). The far less common paralysis of the hand seen after injury to the lower cords of the plexus is named after Klumpke, who described it when she was a medical student. In the great majority of cases the injury causes physiological rather than anatomical interruption of nerve conduction, and spontaneous recovery occurs.

The only other common nerve injury in the newborn is facial palsy. It is a lower motor neurone defect, usually unilateral. It may be associated with, and attributed to, the use of forceps but can occur without. Recovery is the rule.

LOW BIRTH WEIGHT

Babies of low birth weight have special problems and need special care. Terminology is potentially confusing and warrants explanation. Babies with birth weights of 2500 g ($5\frac{1}{2}$ lb) or less, formerly called premature, are now referred to as of low birth weight. Most are born at less than 37 weeks' gestation.

However, birth weight and length of gestation do not always march hand in hand. One baby may weigh less than 2500 g at full term (40 weeks), while a diabetic mother may be delivered at 36 weeks of an infant weighing 4000 g or more. 'Maturity' is a concept which means different things to different people and is not susceptible to precise measurement. Birth weight can be measured accurately and length of gestation reliably in most cases. Babies may be born of low birth weight *either* because their gestation period was cut short, *or* because their intrauterine growth has been retarded. In some infants, both factors operate. We can therefore define two groups of babies requiring special care (Fig. 7).

1   Pre-term babies (less than 37 weeks' gestation). Most will be of low birth weight, but the babies of diabetic and pre-diabetic mothers, however large, face the same problems.

2   Light-for-dates babies (birth weight inappropriately low in relation to the length of gestation). Some authorities prefer the term small-for-dates.

The length of gestation is normally calculated from the first day of the mother's last period and from serial observations of fundal height. In cases of doubt, the biparietal diameter of the fetal skull estimated by ultra-

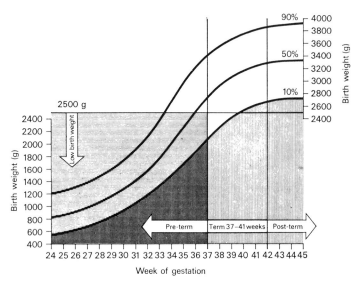

Fig. 7. Pre-term babies (horizontal hatching) are of less than 37 weeks gestation. Light-for-dates babies (vertical hatching) have a weight below the 10% for their gestation.

sound correlates well with gestation. Experimentally, a number of biochemical, cytochemical and cytological tests on amniotic fluid are being developed, which may be helpful in selected cases.

At birth the gestational age of the baby may be estimated from weight, length and head circumference; from certain physical characteristics; by the maturity of the nervous system as assessed by eliciting various reflexes and responses (Fig. 8); and in special cases by assessing biochemical maturity in terms of, for example, immunoglobulins or haemoglobins.

The use of the term 'dysmaturity' to describe certain clinical features exhibited by many light-for-dates babies is discouraged, but will remain in use until a satisfactory alternative has been invented. These features include a lack of subcutaneous fat and dry, wrinkled or cracked skin. 'Postmaturity' should be used, if at all, to mean an excessively long gestation period. 'Placental insufficiency' can only be diagnosed on the basis of placental function tests, of which the most generally used is the maternal urinary excretion of oestriol. Levels which fall, or rise too slowly, with advancing pregnancy strongly suggest impaired placental function.

Pre-term baby (Fig. 9)

The main problems are:
1   feeding;
2   hyperbilirubinaemia;
3   respiratory distress syndrome;
4   infections;
5   brain damage;
6   hypothermia;
7   later, anaemia and vitamin deficiency.

The special problems of *feeding* pre-term babies arise from:
(a) their poorly developed sucking and swallowing reflexes;
(b) the ease with which they regurgitate feeds and may inhale milk, with a risk of inhalation pneumonia;
(c) their large calorie requirement in relation to size.

If sucking and swallowing reflexes are inadequate, or if bottle feeding causes the baby to become exhausted, feeds

Gestation in weeks	< 30	30	31	32	33	34	35	36	37	38	39	40
Physical features — Sole creases	None			Transverse, anterior ⅓					Transverse, anterior ⅔		Criss-cross all over	
Breast nodule	None			Diameter 2 mm					4–5 mm		7–10 mm	
Pinna	Soft, flat, shapeless				Periphery begins to curl					Becoming springy		Difficult to fold
Testes and scrotum	Testes not palpable	Testes in the inguinal canals / Few rugae underside of scrotum						Testes descend into scrotum / Underside of scrotum covered with rugae				
Tone — Posture												
Maximal popliteal angle	180°	160°			150°		120°		100°	90°		< 90°
Reflexes — Pupil response to light	Absent		Present									
Turns to light	Absent							Present				
Sucking					Present							

Fig. 8. Scoring of gestational age.

28

Fig. 9. A pre-term baby of 34 weeks' gestation. She is jaundiced, has prominent labia minora and is lying in a characteristic 'frog's legs' position.

will be given by gastric tube. The risk of regurgitation is minimised by giving small, frequent feeds and reducing the handling of the infant to a minimum. However, to provide adequate calories, the size of the feeds must be increased as rapidly as the infant will tolerate them. Satisfactory weight gain may not be achieved until the infant is receiving as much as 150 cal/kg/day.

Jaundice

Jaundice occurs in all pre-term babies: the more immature the baby, the more marked is the jaundice. This is because the liver enzyme glucuronyl transferase, which is required for the conjugation of bilirubin prior to its excretion, is poorly developed in the newborn, and especially in the pre-term baby. Occasionally bilirubin levels may become dangerously high (250–350 μmol/l or more) with the threat of kernicterus, and exchange transfusion is required. This is more likely to occur if the baby has been hypoxic at any stage or if feeding has been delayed.

The idiopathic respiratory distress syndrome (RDS)

Sometimes called hyaline membrane disease, idiopathic respiratory distress syndrome is a dangerous illness seen only in the newborn period and confined almost entirely to pre-term babies. Affected babies may breathe reasonably well at birth and to the untrained eye may appear to be healthy. Respiration is, however, a little laboured, and becomes progressively more so with the passage of time. Over the course of a few hours respiratory effort increases, but with diminishing effect. With each breath, instead of the lungs expanding, the soft parts of the chest wall sink in so that there is visible recession of the intercostal spaces, the suprasternal fossa and the epigastrium. There may be an audible grunt, and the baby's colour deteriorates. In severe cases there is cyanosis and cardiac failure. Biochemical studies show a profound acidosis, part respiratory and part metabolic, lowered pO_2 and raised pCO_2. The condition proceeds either to death or to complete recovery; sequelae are rare. A chest X-ray shows a granular appearance over the whole of the lungfields. In fatal cases, histological examination of the lungs usually shows an eosinophilic material lining the alveoli and terminal bronchioles (hyaline membrane) which consists largely of fibrin. Chemical examination of the lung fluid shows a marked depletion of surfactant, a lipoprotein normally present in lung fluid and having the property of lowering surface tension and preventing adhesion of alveolar walls. Treatment includes the administration of oxygen, the correction of acidosis by administering intravenous sodium bicarbonate in carefully calculated amounts, the maintenance of calorie intake, and the control of cardiac failure. If respiratory insufficiency is severe and prolonged, assisted ventilation is indicated, but if high concentrations of oxygen or high ventilatory pressures are unavoidable they may cause lung damage (bronchopulmonary dysplasia) which takes weeks to resolve and there is a risk of retrolental fibroplasia leading to blindness. Arterial pO_2 monitoring is essential.

Estimation of lipid content in amniotic fluid (lecithin and sphyngomyelin) provides a good guide to the development of surfactant and the risk of respiratory distress. When early induction of labour is planned, this test can help in deciding the best time for the baby. The incidence of RDS is significantly reduced if women in premature labour are given glucocorticoids.

Respiratory distress may also occur in pneumonia, with pulmonary haemorrhage and in babies with brain damage.

Infections

The liability of the pre-term infant to infections is largely determined by the immaturity of his humoral immunity. The greatest risk is from gram-negative bacterial infections, especially pneumonia, septicaemia and meningitis. Further details are given on page 38.

Brain damage

The pre-term brain is a very soft organ, almost fluid, and the blood vessels within and around it have very delicate walls. The forces to which the fetal skull and its contents are exposed in normal labour may be sufficient to cause brain damage in the small baby: difficult labour is even more hazardous. The obstetrician minimizes the trauma by carrying out episiotomy and delivering the baby with extra care. Risks to the brain after birth include hyperbilirubinaemia, hypoglycaemia and meningitis. Earlier follow-up studies of pre-term babies, especially those of very low birth weight, revealed a depressingly high incidence of physical and mental defect. More recent studies from modern neonatal units providing comprehensive monitoring, show more encouraging results, the

31

incidence of handicap being scarcely greater than in full-term babies.

Hypothermia

Pre-term babies have a poorly developed temperature-regulating mechanism and easily cool. Nursing in an incubator permits accurate control of ambient air temperature and humidity together with unimpeded observation. Heat loss can be further reduced by wrapping the baby in aluminium foil ('silver swaddler').

Anaemia

Pre-term babies often develop quite severe anaemia when 2 or 3 months old. The aetiology is complex. The anaemia can usually be prevented by giving prophylactic iron supplements, or will respond to iron if it has developed. The deficiency arises from the disparity between the iron intake and the very rapid rate of growth, with a correspondingly rapid increase in blood volume. Sometimes the anaemia is megaloblastic and responds to folic acid. In a few pre-term babies anaemia is evident much earlier and results from temporary marrow hypoplasia. The rapid rate of growth also renders pre-term babies more prone to vitamin-deficiency diseases. It is therefore advisable that all pre-term babies should be given supplements of vitamins as well as iron until their diets contain adequate amounts (6–9 months).

Light-for-dates baby (Fig. 10)

The special problems of the light-for-dates baby are:
1 hypoglycaemia;
2 skin infection;
3 poor post-natal growth.

Neonatal hypoglycaemia

The normal blood glucose level in the newborn is low in comparison to older infants. Symptoms are rarely seen unless the level falls below 1.0 mmol/l. The symptoms are irritability, pallor and reluctance with feeds. Frank

Fig. 10. Two babies born at 40 weeks' gestation. That on the left weighs a normal 3·5 kg. That on the right is light-for-dates, weighing 2 kg; he is thin and has a dry wrinkled skin.

twitching proceeding to generalised convulsions occurs later. There is a danger that hypoglycaemia may cause brain damage and, therefore, on the least suspicion the blood glucose level should be checked. The best way to prevent neonatal hypoglycaemia is early feeding. Mild hypoglycaemia may be treated by frequent feeds with added glucose; more severe forms require intravenous glucose.

Skin infection

The dry, cracked skin of the light-for-dates baby renders it especially prone to skin infection with staphylococci. Infections are best treated by antiseptic creams.

Slow growth

Most light-for-dates babies are hungry and gain weight well. A few behave as if permanently adjusted to slow growth. They feed poorly from birth and appear to have small food requirements. They grow slowly, and their weight and height increase parallel to, but below, the 3rd centile on growth charts. Some of these infants have one or both parents well below average size. Bone age is usually retarded and epiphyses fuse relatively late, so there is an opportunity for some catch-up growth at puberty. As growth patterns are largely determined very early in life, every effort should be made to achieve good weight gain in the neonatal period.

JAUNDICE IN THE NEWBORN

Jaundice is extremely common in newborn infants and is usually noted on the 2nd and 3rd day of life, gradually fading over the next few days. This is *physiological jaundice* and results from a temporary inadequacy of bilirubin glucuronyl transferase in the liver. This is especially marked in pre-term babies virtually all of whom develop jaundice. Physiological jaundice may be protracted in cretins, and this may be the first diagnostic clue. In healthy, full-term babies bilirubin levels in physiological jaundice rarely exceed 200 μmol/l. In small pre-term babies higher levels may be reached with the risk of kernicterus (p. 36). In these infants phototherapy with blue light may prevent bilirubin levels becoming dangerously high, but exchange tranfusion is sometimes needed.

Jaundice appearing in the first 24 hours of life is never physiological. It is more often due to haemolytic disease than to all other causes. The more common causes of neonatal jaundice are shown in Table 4.

Table 4. Causes of neonatal jaundice

Type of jaundice	Causes
Bilirubin largely unconjugated	Physiological jaundice
	Haemolytic disease (rhesus, ABO, etc.)
	Other haemolytic anaemias (hereditary spherocytocis: G6PD deficiency)
	After extensive internal bleeding (especially cephalhaematoma)
Bilirubin mixed	Sepsis (septicaemia or other severe infection)
	Neonatal hepatitis
	Galactosaemia
Bilirubin largely conjugated	Biliary atresia

Haemolytic disease of the newborn

A woman may become sensitized to red cell antigens either as a result of fetal red cells leaking across the placental barrier, usually at the end of a pregnancy, or as a consequence of the transfusion of improperly matched blood. If, in her next pregnancy, the fetus has the same red cell antigen, maternal antibody will cross the placenta and begin to destroy fetal red cells. This is haemolytic disease, and most commonly occurs in a rhesus positive infant whose rhesus negative mother has become sensitized to the D rhesus antigen. Less commonly, haemolytic disease results from incompatibility of other rhesus antigens, ABO antigens, or the rare blood group antigens. Haemolysis leads to anaemia, the severity of which depends upon the rate of red cell destruction and the efficiency with which new red cells are produced. There is very active erythropoiesis in the liver and spleen as well as in the marrow, and primitive red cells—reticulocytes, normoblasts, erythroblasts—are plentiful in the peripheral blood: hence the alternative name, erythroblastosis fetalis. In the most severe cases, the profound anaemia leads to fetal heart failure with gross oedema (hydrops fetalis) which carries a very high mortality rate.

Bilirubin conjugation and excretion are carried on fairly efficiently by the fetus in utero. The amniotic fluid is bile-stained, but the serum bilirubin level of cord blood is never more than 100 μmol/l unless there is an element of obstructive jaundice (inspissated bile syndrome). After birth, however, the bilirubin level begins to climb and clinical jaundice becomes evident or more marked within a few hours of birth. Haemolytic disease is by far the most common cause of jaundice noticed within 24 hours of birth in Caucasian infants. Because of the relative inefficiency of the neonatal liver, especially in pre-term babies, the serum bilirubin level may reach 350–500 μmol/l or more. This is predominantly unconjugated bilirubin which is soluble in lipid but not in water (it has to be fat-soluble before birth in order to cross the placenta). If the level is allowed to rise too high, bilirubin may be deposited in the grey matter of the brain, especially the basal ganglia, causing kernicterus. This is the most dangerous complication of haemolytic disease, leading to death or to survival with permanent brain damage. Clinically, it presents with irritability, poor feeding, head retraction, down-turned eyes ('setting sun sign') and convulsions. Late sequelae include mental defect, cerebral palsy (athetoid or spastic) and perceptive deafness.

Haemolytic disease is preventable unless the mother has already developed antibodies. The initial sensitizing event virtually always occurs around the time of birth (or abortion) of a rhesus positive baby. If anti-D immunoglobulin is given to all rhesus negative women by intravenous injection shortly after delivery (birth or abortion) any D positive cells in her circulation (fetal cells) will be destroyed before the mother has begun to develop any antibodies to them. Any remaining injected antibody is eliminated very quickly.

For those women who already have antibodies, prevention is not possible. All their rhesus positive babies will be affected. The clinical picture at birth varies from the mildest with no abnormal signs, through moderate with definite pallor and some enlargement of the liver and spleen, to severe with profound anaemia, marked hepatosplenomegaly and perhaps jaundice. The direct Coombs' test is positive, and the haemoglobin and bilirubin levels in cord blood give a useful indication of the severity of the disease. Midly affected infants require no treatment at birth. The haemoglobin will fall over the next 6–8 weeks;

if it drops below 7 g/dl, simple transfusion is advisable. More severe cases require transfusion earlier and perhaps more than once. The most severe cases, as judged by clinical and laboratory findings, and in the light of the history of previously affected children, may require exchange transfusion. This procedure replaces most of the infant's blood with donor rhesus negative blood (which will not be destroyed by antibody), raises the haemoglobin level, and removes most of the doomed rhesus positive cells together with some circulating bilirubin. In a few infants more than one exchange transfusion may be necessary.

A severely affected infant may not survive to full term, and a decision may have to be made to deliver the infant earlier. The hazards of immaturity are then added to those of haemolytic disease, and the decision calls for experience and judgement.

Only haemolytic disease due to D antigen will be anticipated by routine antenatal blood tests. The remaining cases will only be recognised when an infant develops jaundice within 24 hours of birth. ABO incompatibility most commonly occurs in a group A baby of a group O mother. It is usually mild. Rare blood group incompatibilities can only be diagnosed by special haematological investigation, and it may be difficult to find suitable donor blood for exchange transfusion.

OTHER NEONATAL PROBLEMS

Haemorrhagic disease of the newborn

Just as the liver of the newborn baby, and especially of the pre-term baby, takes a few days to become competent at conjugating bilirubin, so it is temporarily inefficient at synthesizing many blood clotting factors. Serial measurements of the prothrombin level, for example, will usually show a fall from cord blood levels until about the third day of life, after which it improves, reaching normal levels about 7–10 days after birth. In the great majority of infants there are no clinical symptoms, but occasionally there is spontaneous bleeding, usually from the gastrointestinal tract, on the 2nd or 3rd day of life. Melaena is recognisable by a dark red tinge to the meconium;

vomited blood is usually dark brown. The amount of blood lost is rarely enough to disturb health, but occasionally there is sufficient blood loss to necessitate transfusion. Otherwise treatment comprises the intramuscular injection of vitamin K_1, 1 mg, repeated if necessary.

Pre-term and anoxic infants are more prone to develop haemorrhagic disease than healthy, full-term babies. Prophylactic vitamin K_1 may be given at birth to infants at particular risk, but some paediatricians prefer every infant to receive it.

Deficiency of clotting factors may also contribute to bleeding from the umbilicus or into the subaponeurotic space of the scalp. The latter is much more serious than cephalhaematoma (p. 24), because the extent of the bleeding is almost unlimited and the baby may become exsanguinated with alarming rapidity. Other causes of neonatal gastrointestinal bleeding include:

1   Swallowed maternal blood, either
    (a) following antepartum or intrapartum haemorrhage, or
    (b) as a result of feeding from engorged breasts.
Large amounts of blood may be vomited, but the baby shows no signs of blood loss. If the blood has not become denatured in the stomach, maternal blood can be distinguished chemically from infant's blood.

2   Hiatus hernia. The predominant feature is vomiting; there may be a little altered blood, but frank melaena is rare.

Infections

Some babies are born infected, some acquire infection during birth, and some have infection thrust upon them after birth. The principal infections in each category are as follows:

1   Acquired before birth:
    (a) cytomegalovirus
    (b) rubella
    (c) toxoplasmosis
    (d) syphilis
    (e) hepatitis B
    (f) varicella/herpes

2   Acquired during birth:
    (a) gonorrhoea
    (b) moniliasis
3   Acquired after birth:
    (a) staphylococcal infections of the skin, umbilicus, eye or nail-bed.
    (b) gram-negative bacterial infections (commonly *Escherichia coli*)—septicaemia, meningitis, pneumonia, urinary tract infections.
    (c) group B haemolytic streptococci

Infection of a developing embryo is likely to cause death and abortion. The *rubella* virus, although undoubtedly capable of causing embryonic death, also has the unique ability to cause malformations compatible with life, notably congenital heart disease, cataract and other eye defects, perceptive deafness, and microcephaly with mental retardation. In addition, an infected baby may be born with evidence of active viraemia as shown by jaundice, hepatosplenomegaly, purpura and sometimes lesions of the bones and lungs (Fig. 11). This 'extended rubella syndrome' can occur without malformations. A baby with congenital rubella has persisting endogenous antibody and may also excrete live virus from the pharynx and the kidneys for as long as 2 years. Congenital rubella may be confirmed by isolation of virus from throat washings or urine, by demonstrating specific rubella IgM in the baby, or by persistence of rubella antibody after the age of 8 months.

Hepatitis is a conspicuous feature of other intrauterine infections, the liver being the first organ reached by blood from the placenta. Jaundice and hepatomegaly are therefore common presenting features. In congenital syphilis, which is very rare in Britain now, skin rashes and snuffles may be present at birth. Infection with *Toxoplasma gondii* or *cytomegalovirus* (CMV) may damage the central nervous system or eye, resulting in mental retardation, epilepsy, microcephaly, hydrocephalus, microphthalmia or choroiditis. These diagnoses are confirmed by serological tests on infants and mother. Prenatal infection with CMV is commoner than congenital rubella, but most infected babies are clinically normal.

The common '*sticky eye*' is essentially a drainage problem. If tears cannot drain adequately down the

Fig. 11. Features of the rubella syndrome.

Cataract
Glaucoma
Microphthalmia
Chorioretinitis

Bulging fontanelle
Encephalopathy
Mental retardation
Microcephaly
Perceptive deafness

Congenital
heart disease:
P.D.A.
P.S.
VSD/ASD
myocarditis
Pneumonitis
Thrombocytopaenic
purpura

Hepatosplenomegaly
Jaundice

Also abortion and
stillbirth in pregnancy
Low birth weight

Osteolytic lesions

nasolacrymal duct they tend to pool in the inner canthus in the supine infant. In this pool the ubiquitous staphylococcus multiplies, producing a small amount of pus which dries. The conjunctivae remain clear. The condition subsides within 2–3 weeks. Secretions can be gently bathed away as necessary: antibiotics, though often used, are only necessary in severe cases. By contrast, gonococcal ophthalmia, which was once the commonest cause of blindness in children, is now rare. There is much periorbital oedema which makes it difficult to open the eyes. If the lids are forced apart, copious creamy pale yellow pus wells out. Vigorous treatment is needed with an antibiotic to which the organism is sensitive.

Oral thrush (moniliasis) present within a few days of birth is often the result of a maternal infection of the genital tract. If the infection develops later, it is more likely to have been acquired from unsterilized dummies, teats or bottles. The source of infection should be traced if possible and dealt with by treatment or advice. Nystatin suspension should be applied to the mouth lesions after feeds. Monilial infections in other sites are rare in the newborn period.

Escherichia coli is the most dangerous organism to the newborn baby. It may cause septicaemia, meningitis, pneumonia, urinary infections or gastroenteritis. It can probably be acquired either during or after birth and is responsible for most of the serious and lethal infections of the neonate. Whereas the alimentary tract of the breast-fed baby is colonised by lactobacilli, in the bottle-fed baby *E. coli* is predominant. The early signs of infection in the newborn are inconspicuous and will only be detected by the experienced and vigilant eye. A reluctance to feed, a slightly loose stool, slight vomiting, unsatisfactory weight gain, a cyanotic attack, irritability or a small flick of temperature may be the first hint of trouble. Later, vomiting, diarrhoea, weight loss, fever, convulsions, jaundice or rash make it obvious that the baby is ill. There is often little in the way of localizing symptoms or signs. Blood culture, lumbar puncture, chest X-ray and urine examination will be needed, but if clinical suspicions exist, parenteral antibiotics must be started without waiting for laboratory reports. The longer the delay, the greater the risk of death or brain damage. Amongst the many antibiotic regimes advocated, penicillin or ampicillin together with gentamicin are widely used.

Staphylococcal infections are very common but rarely severe. Sticky eyes, septic spots, sticky umbilicus and paronychia will respond to simple local measures. More severe skin infections require systemic antibiotics (e.g. cloxacillin). *Beta-haemolytic streptococci* of Lancefield group B are responsible for an increasing number of septicaemic and pneumonic infections in the newborn, the latter clinically resembling hyaline membrane disease.

Hypocalcaemia

Hypocalcaemic tetany characteristically occurs in

bottle-fed babies about a week old. It presents with localised twitchings, especially of the hands and feet, or with generalised convulsions. The serum calcium is usually below 1·8 μmol/l, and this may be partly due to the high phosphate content of cow's milk in comparison with human milk. It is rarely seen in babies fed on low-solute milks. Mild cases are treated with oral calcium supplements and sedation, more severe cases with parenteral calcium. The convulsions usually respond readily and the long-term prognosis is good. Less frequently hypocalcaemia arises in the first 3 days of life: the reason for this is obscure.

Occasionally hypocalcaemia fails to respond to adequate doses of calcium. It may then be found that the serum magnesium is below the normal 0·5–1 μmol/l. Intramuscular magnesium sulphate is effective treatment. Hypomagnesaemia without hypocalcaemia is excessively rare.

Convulsions

Convulsions are always a serious symptom and nowhere more so than in the neonatal period. The cause must be determined and, if possible, treated. Most seizures will respond to phenobarbitone or chloral hydrate unless there is severe brain damage. The main causes of neonatal convulsions have been described in this chapter, and are summarized below:
1   Brain damage:
    (a) physical—intracranial haemorrhage,
    (b) chemical—hypoxia
                  kernicterus.
2   Infections:
    (a) septicaemia,
    (b) meningitis.
3   Metabolic disorders:
    (a) hypoglycaemia,
    (b) hypocalcaemia.
Fits in the first 48 hours carry the poorest prognosis. Between one-third and one-half of affected babies die. Fits which occur later in the neonatal period are rarely associated with death or serious handicap.

Further reading

Chiswick M. *Neonatal Medicine*. Update Publications.

Cockburn F. & Drillien C. M. *Neonatal Medicine*. Blackwell Scientific Publications.

Norman A. P. *Congenital Abnormalities in Infancy*. Blackwell Scientific Publications.

Schaffer A. J. and Avery M. A. *Diseases of the Newborn*. W. B. Saunders.

Vulliamy D.C. *The Newborn Child*. Churchill-Livingstone.

Chapter 3

Infant Feeding

Babies treble their birth weight in the first year of life; to treble it again takes 10 years. Furthermore, 65% of total post-natal brain growth takes place in the first year of life. Nutrition is therefore more important in infancy than at any other age. Starvation may permanently hamper both physical and mental development. Average nutritional requirements in infancy are:

Water	150 ml/kg/day ($2\frac{1}{2}$ oz/lb/day);
Calories	110 cal/kg/day (50 cal/lb/day);
Vitamin C	15 mg/day;
Vitamin D	400 i.u./day (10 μg cholecalciferol);
Calcium	600 mg/day ⎫
Iron	6 mg/day ⎬ average during first year.

MILK

Milk is a poor source of iron but rich in calcium and calories. There is little fat-soluble vitamin D in human milk, but substantial amounts of water-soluble vitamin D sulphate. The main differences in composition between human and cow's milk are shown below:

	Human milk (per 100 ml)		Cow's milk (per 100 ml)	
Protein	1·2 g		3·3 g	
Casein	0·3 g		2·7 g	
Soluble proteins	0·9 g		0·6 g	
Lactose	7·0 g		4·8 g	
Fat	3·7 g		3·7 g	
Saturated		48%		58%
Unsaturated		52%		42%
Sodium	15 mg		58 mg	
Phosphorus	15 mg		100 mg	

It will be noted that in cow's milk the protein content is much higher and most of it is casein: the lactose content is lower: the fat content is similar, but more of it is in the form of saturated fatty acids. The sodium (and potassium) content is higher, leading to a higher osmolality. The phosphorus content is higher. The processing of cow's milk alters the protein so that reconstituted dried or evaporated milks are more easily digested by infants than is fresh cow's milk. Doorstep milk should not be given to infants under 6 months. From 6 to 12 months of age it may be given, but it must be boiled first if (a) it is not pasteurised, (b) home conditions are poor or (c) there is no refrigerator.

Strenuous attempts have been made to formulate infant feeds to approximate closely to breast milk in regard to protein, lactose, fat, sodium and phosphorus content. These modern milks are fortified with vitamin D, and some with vitamin C and iron (the bioavailability of this iron is not as good as that in breast milk).

A *full-strength* feed is made up according to the instructions on the container; a *half-strength* feed is made up with double the usual amount of water.

BREAST FEEDING

Successful breast feeding requires the active partici-
pation of both parties. The baby needs well-established sucking and swallowing reflexes and a good appetite. These are normally present in the healthy, full-term infant but may be defective in the sick or pre-term infant. The mother needs a good draught reflex, which may take a little while to develop with a first baby. The stimulus to this reflex initially is contact of the baby with the nipple, but later the baby's hunger cry, or even thinking about the baby, may be sufficient. The response is a secretion by the posterior pituitary of oxytocin which causes contraction of the myoepithelial cells around the alveoli of the breast, with ejection of milk down the ducts to the ampulla. In the puerperium, the oxytocin secreted will also cause uterine contraction, and midwives tradi-
tionally used to put the newborn baby straight to the breast to encourage expulsion of the placenta. For the

same reason, breast feeding may be associated with abdominal cramps in the first week or two.

Breast-fed babies may be fed by the clock (usually every 4 hours) or on demand. Regular weighing is the only means of knowing whether the milk supply is adequate. Crying does not necessarily mean hunger; sleep does not necessarily mean satiation. Breast feeding can be a highly satisfying experience for the mother and ensures close physical contact between mother and infant. There is, however, no evidence to suggest that bottle-fed babies are either nutritionally or emotionally deprived. Infant feeding practices seem to be dictated largely by fashion. Mothers may feel that breast feeding limits their social activities, spoils their clothes or ruins their figures. Rich families in past ages employed wet nurses (e.g. Exodus, 2, vii): today the bottle is more readily available. There are many good reasons for encouraging mothers to breast feed, and the encouragement should start no later than the antenatal clinic. Breast milk is nutritionally ideal for at least 4 months in the full-term baby. It is inexpensive, readily available, and convenient. Breast-fed babies are less prone to gastroenteritis, infantile eczema, obesity, hypocalcaemic fits and hypernatraemic states.

Protection from infection results not only from the reduced opportunity to contaminate the milk. Maternal antibody in breast milk discourages colonisation of the gut by pathogens. The pH of breast milk and the presence of certain substances, including lactoferrin and bifidus factor, encourage colonisation of the bowel with lactobacilli rather than coliforms. Breast feeding, even for a month, gives an infant an excellent start to life. Nobody wants to see unwilling mothers browbeaten into breast feeding, but there is a happy mean between that and the total indifference shown by many doctors and nurses. Experience has shown repeatedly that mothers will respond to information, advice and encouragement.

BOTTLE FEEDING

Bottle feeding offers opportunities to infect the baby, and the preparation of feeds and sterilization of bottles must therefore be meticulous. Bottles and teats may be sterilized by boiling or by immersion in hypochlorite solution:

by either method, attention to detail is crucial. Evaporated milks are sterile, and dried milks pathogen-free,
until the tins are opened. Feeds should normally be made
up according to the manufacturer's directions and should
be given either 4-hourly or on demand. The newborn baby
will require feeding round the clock, but within a few
weeks will drop the night feed. So long as a night feed is
demanded, it must be given. Leaving him to cry is
pointless and unkind.

Attention to detail in making up the feed is as essential
as detail in sterilizing bottles. The scoop appropriate to
the milk powder should be used, it should be filled without
compressing the powder (unless otherwise stated) and
should be levelled off with a knife. Additional scoops,
heaped scoops, packed scoops or additional cereal should
be avoided. They add extra calories which encourage
obesity, and extra solutes which cause thirst and irritability.

MIXED FEEDING

The age at which foods other than milk are introduced
has been influenced to some extent by fashion. A full-term
baby will not develop any nutritional deficiency within 4
months of birth, and this is the earliest age at which
mixed feeding should start. Pre-term infants grow faster
than full-term babies and should be given iron and
vitamin supplements until they are taking a mixed diet.
The main principles of mixed feeding are:

1   Ensure an adequate introduction of food containing
protein and iron; avoid *excess* carbohydrate (e.g. cereals).

2   Introduce one new food at a time, starting with very
small quantities and increasing gradually if the food is
accepted and tolerated.

3   If a new food is not accepted by the infant, try
something else. Later feeding difficulties may stem from
misguided insistence on an infant taking food that he
does not enjoy.

As the semi-solid component of the diet is increased, the
number and volume of milk feeds should be decreased.
The duration of breast feeding rarely exceeds 3 months in
Western societies, but averages 2 years or more in
developing countries. The average 1-year-old will be

having three main meals a day, with a small drink or snack mid-morning, mid-afternoon and at bedtime.

FEEDING PROBLEMS

Difficulties with feeding are common. In very young infants they may be to do with bottles, but at all ages they are more likely to do with battles. Feeding mismanagement in early life may present with vomiting, disturbed bowel habit, unsatisfactory weight gain or crying. Most difficulties arise from one or more of three faults.

1   The *quantity* of food is wrong. Both underfeeding and overfeeding may lead to vomiting and crying. In the first, weight gain is consistently poor. An overfed baby gains weight excessively to begin with, but may later lose. Overfeeding is particularly common in bottle-fed babies, partly because they are often fed to the limit of their capacity, partly because food has a sedative effect, and partly because of the mistaken belief that the biggest babies are the best.

2   The *kind* of food is wrong. Excessively early mixed feeding may lead to vomiting, diarrhoea and crying. A return to a milk diet will allow recovery, followed by a more cautious weaning programme. Changing from one milk to another rarely achieves anything.

3   The feeding *technique* is wrong. This is a common cause of difficulties and can only be recognized by watching the baby feeding. The baby may not be held comfortably; the bottle may be held at the wrong angle; the hole in the teat may be too small or too big; the milk may have been wrongly prepared. Instruction and advice provide the remedy.

One particular form of crying in early infancy deserves special mention. *Three-months colic*, or evening colic, is a very common problem arising in early life and lasting, as a rule, not beyond the age of 3 months. An otherwise placid baby devotes one part of the day, most commonly between the 6 p.m. and 10 p.m. feeds, to incessant crying. He may or may not stop when picked up, but certainly cries again if put down. Attention to feeds, warmth, wet nappies, etc. are unavailing. Theories abound but the cause is unknown. Many such infants derive relief from dicyclomine syrup, 5 ml, at the appropriate time of day.

Dr Benjamin Spock, whose writings have probably had more influence on child rearing than any since Dr Truby King, suggests that at any feed an infant needs to achieve a certain amount of food and a certain amount of sucking. Babies vary in their need for sucking time. Most babies take a feed in 20–30 minutes, but some drain their bottle in 5–10 minutes and may then have filled their stomachs without satisfying their need to suck. Such an infant may solve his own problems by discovering how to suck his thumb. The widespread use of comforters (dummies) in the face of sometimes vehement opposition from the medical and nursing professions suggests that mothers have known this for a long time. Since comforters will continue to be used, just as fireworks will continue to be made and sold, it may be more constructive to stop trying to abolish them and instead try to ensure that they are used safely. Their only hazard is as a vehicle for infection: they do not make teeth protrude. By contrast, the devices consisting of a teat attached to a small reservoir designed to hold sweet fluids have been shown conclusively to dissolve away incisor teeth with startling efficiency and should be condemned outright.

Feeding difficulties after 6 months may result from allowing unsuitable foods, but with increasing age they more commonly result from attempts to insist on the child eating foods which he dislikes. There is a delicate distinction between encouraging the conservative child to try something new, and coercing the reluctant child to eat 'what is good to him'. The mother who sits by the high chair supplying endless diversions whilst she subtly spoons in 'one for Sarah, one for Teddy', is more likely to be storing up trouble than solving a problem. The management of such problems lies in the patient, repeated but firm explanation that no normal child with access to food will starve; that children of some ages are dominated by the need for food, but at other ages it may be a low priority; that wise parents do not start battles with their children that they are bound to lose; and that a mother will often achieve most by doing least.

Some groups of children present inherent problems with feeding. Pre-term babies make no demands and must be fed by the clock. Some mentally retarded children are also abnormally placid and cannot be demand fed: they may also have sucking and swallowing difficulties. Physically handicapped children, especially those with cerebral palsy, may be very difficult to feed because of muscular weakness and incoordination.

Further reading

Mac Keith R. & Wood C. *Infant Feeding and Feeding Difficulties.* J. & A. Churchill.

Chapter 4

Growth and Development

The characteristics of children which most clearly distinguish them from adults are that they are growing and developing. Adults are not growing, except perhaps in girth, and most of them are degenerating. The processes of growth and development start from conception and are influenced by a wide variety of genetic and environmental variables. Growth may be affected by disease: it may also affect the manifestations of disease. For example, if the aqueduct of Sylvius is blocked in an infant, the head will enlarge (hydrocephalus) but the intracranial pressure may not rise very much. If the same event occurs in an older child, the head will not enlarge but the intracranial pressure will rise rapidly.

PHYSICAL GROWTH

Growth is traditionally estimated by weight and height (length in babies) and this is sufficient for most purposes. In clinical medicine other measurements, including sitting height (which reflects body proportions, Fig. 12), span, skinfold thicknesses, and skeletal age by X-ray (p. 54), may be needed to elucidate particular problems. Growth and development are not necessarily smooth, continuous processes. Weight and height increase relatively rapidly in the early months of life and at puberty, but at a very constant rate between. The circumference of the head does half its total growing in the first year of life. Sexual development is concentrated into two episodes, at the 6th week of embryonic life and at puberty.

When interpreting measurements of growth and development it is important to distinguish between normal and average. It is useful to known the average weight of a 1-year-old, the average age at which a child walks

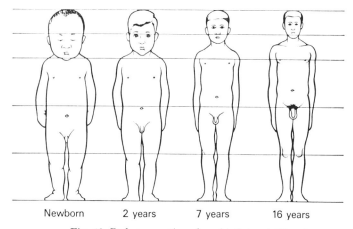

Fig. 12. Body proportions from birth to adulthood.

unaided, and the average head circumference of a newborn baby. It is also vital to know how far removed from
average a measurement can be and yet remain within the
range of normal. For each parameter there is a distribution curve, and this can be indicated on standard record
charts by showing centiles (percentiles) or standard
deviations as well as averages (Fig. 13). The 3rd and 97th
centiles approximate to ± 2 standard deviations. About
3% of normal children will be below the 3rd centile and
another 3% above the 97th centile. In normally propor-
tioned children, whether large, average or small for their
age, the height and weight will occupy similar positions
on centile charts. Much more can be learned from serial
observations of height, weight or head circumference
than from a single measurement. The normal ranges for
these are given in Appendixes 1, 2 and 3.

The potential for physical growth after birth is determined largely by genetic factors. The extent to which this
potential is achieved may be influenced by nutrition, by
disease, and probably also by emotional factors. Failure
of normal physical growth is usually recognized in
infants by unsatisfactory weight gain (failure to thrive)
and in older children by short stature. Sometimes weight
gain is excessive (obesity) and very rarely height may
increase abnormally rapidly.

Fig. 13. A growth record (centile chart) for height. The records contain a similar chart for weight, and are available to cover the age ranges 0–3, 2–10, and 9–18 years for each sex.

Bone age (or skeletal age) is a useful parameter of growth and is determined from X-rays, of the hand and wrist at most ages, though the knee and foot are helpful in small babies. The bones and epiphyses calcify, and hence become visible on X-rays, in a regular order. Later the epiphyses fuse in a similar regular fashion. X-rays can be compared with age-related standards (as in the Greulich and Pyle atlas, based on American children) or can be scored by more complex methods such as the British Tanner and Whitehouse scheme. In healthy children bone age relates more closely to height than to age, short children tending to have 'delayed', and tall children 'advanced' bone age. Bone age is strikingly delayed in hypothyroidism and hypopituitarism: it may be advanced in hyperadrenocorticism and hyperthyroidism.

Failure to thrive

The term is applied to a child in the first year or two of life whose predominant symptom is unsatisfactory weight gain. The main causes are:
1   Inadequate food intake
    (a) Feeding mismanagement or neglect,
    (b) Poor appetite,
    (c) Mechanical problems, e.g. cleft palate, cerebral palsy.
2   Vomiting
    (a) Pyloric stenosis, hiatus hernia,
    (b) Feeding mismanagement.
3   Defects of digestion or absorption
    (a) Cystic fibrosis,
    (b) Coeliac disease,
    (c) Chronic infective diarrhoea.
4   Failure of utilization
    (a) Chronic infections (especially urinary),
    (b) Heart failure, renal failure,
    (c) Metabolic disorders.
5   Emotional deprivation
In the majority of instances a diagnosis will be reached on the basis of a detailed history and full examination including watching the baby feed and testing the urine.

Short stature

The majority of children for whom medical advice is sought because of short stature are normal, short children. Some of them were born light-for-dates and many have short relatives including one or both parents. Their *rate* of growth is normal, as shown by serial measurements plotted on a centile chart. Most of these children have delayed skeletal development, their pubertal growth spurt is often late and they continue growing for longer than the average. If serial observations of height show an abnormally slow rate of increase, some other explanation must be sought. The main causes of pathological short stature are:

1   Defects of nutrition, digestion or absorption (p. 178).
2   Chronic disease.
3   Disorders of bone growth (e.g. achondroplasia).
4   Deficiency of thyroid or growth hormone.
5   Protracted steroid therapy.
6   Most malformation syndromes.
7   Social and emotional deprivation.

Thyroid deficiency in infancy is likely to be recognized from other symptoms and signs before short stature becomes apparent (p. 242). Growth hormone deficiency may be isolated or may be part of a wider pituitary insufficiency. Growth hormone response to exercise or hypoglycaemia may be measured. The ratio of the upper body segment to the lower is normal for the age in hypopituitarism: in hypothyroidism the proportions tend to remain infantile. Skeletal development is retarded in both conditions but especially in hypothyroidism.

If the cause of short stature can be removed or corrected, catch-up growth to expected height is often achieved over some years.

Excessive stature

Excessive stature is only rarely due to disturbed pituitary function. Usually it is due to genetic factors, the tall child having tall relatives. Rarer causes include Marfan's syndrome. The prediction of ultimate height is difficult, but if it seems likely that it will exceed acceptable limits the epiphyses at the knee may be fused by operation. Hormone therapy is of doubtful benefit.

Chromosome anomalies often affect stature, children with Down's and Turner's syndromes being short and some with Klinefelter's syndrome tall.

Obesity

Obesity in childhood is a common and troublesome problem—troublesome to the child, the family and the doctor. Some heavyweight newborns seem to have insatiable appetites, their price for peace is food, and they seem doomed to obesity from the womb (Fig. 14). In others, the

Fig. 14. An obese 3-month-old baby weighing 8·2 kg.

tendency to excessive weight gain may appear in infancy, toddlerhood or during school years. Although only 10–20% of obese infants are still fat when they start school, half of all fat schoolchildren were overweight as babies. Fat children often come from fat families. Many fat children are undoubtedly gluttons, tucking away excessive calories, predominantly from carbohydrates. Equally certainly, some fat children do not eat excessively but have an abnormal tendency to lay down fat. Similarly, some fat children take a lot of exercise, others none. Obese children are nearly always tall for their age. Obesity combined with short stature suggests a possible endocrine cause.

Obesity may limit exercise tolerance; associated knock knee may lead to complaints of leg pains; and in boys the disappearance of the penis into a pad of suprapubic fat may lead to a mistaken diagnosis of hypogonadism. The dominant symptoms, however, are psychological. The fat child may be teased and ostracized, and the fat girl cannot buy fashionable clothes. There is good evidence that fat children tend to become fat adults, and weight reduction is advisable. The patients (especially boys) and their families are often ambivalent about dieting: they would like to lose weight, but not with sufficient zeal to endure the inconvenience.

For most children, a 1000 calorie diet, encouragement to exercise, and ample moral support form the basis of treatment. Group activities may help. Drugs are best avoided; amphetamines should not be prescribed. Any emotional stresses at home or at school should if possible be alleviated. If satisfactory weight loss is achieved, follow-up should not be too short. If necessary, admission to hospital allows the strict supervision of a more restricted diet and weight is rapidly lost. Sadly, it is often regained rapidly after returning home. Finally, obesity is **almost never due to endocrine disease and parents need to be told that the child's 'glands are alright'.**

DEFECTIVE NUTRITION

Nutritional deficiency may consist in a general shortage of food or in lack of specific dietary factors. Overall food deficiency is only seen in Britain in children who have been grossly neglected, but in many parts of the world, especially the tropics and subtropics, *infantile marasmus* is all too common. In these areas, breast-feeding is customarily continued for about 2 years, and there is very little alternative. If the supply of breast milk is inadequate, starvation ensues. The infant with marasmus is a prey to intercurrent infection, and mortality is high. There is also evidence that starvation in the first year of life, even if subsequently corrected, may cause permanent mental handicap.

Kwashiorkor, or protein–calorie malnutrition, is seen in the same parts of the world as marasmus but in older children, usually 2–4 years old. At this age the next baby often displaces the older sibling from the breast, and in many places it is customary to send the older child away to stay with relatives after the new baby has arrived. Food deprivation may therefore coincide with emotional disturbance, and the characteristic picture of kwashiorkor develops. The child is listless, the face, limbs and abdomen swell, the hair is sparse and dry, and there are areas of hyperpigmentation ('black enamel paint') especially on the legs. Diarrhoea is sometimes a feature.

An increasing number of Western families are adopting bizarre diets in the name of religion or conservation. Growing children fed on such diets may be malnourished.

Rickets

Nutritional rickets results from dietary deficiency of vitamin D coupled with inadequate exposure to sunlight. It is quite common in Asian children in the U.K. because their traditional diet is poor in calcium and they receive little sunlight on their skins. Rickets may complicate malabsorption states and certain rare forms of renal disease. Normal bone formation requires a proper balance of calcium and phosphorus in the tissues, especially at the epiphyses where active growth is most rapid. Vitamin D is involved in the absorption of calcium from the gut and in the deposition of normal bone. Deficiency of calcium, phosphorus or vitamin D interfere with bone maturation beyond the stage of provisional calcification which therefore tends to accumulate as osteoid tissue. This accounts for the thickening of epiphyses seen particularly at the wrists, ankles and costo-chondral junctions ('rickety rosary'). The frontal bones may also be thickened. Toddlers develop bow legs: older children become knock-kneed. There is hypotonia.

In nutritional rickets the serum calcium is normal or reduced and the alkaline phosphatase is raised. X-rays show broadening, cupping and rarefaction of the bone ends (Fig. 15). In malabsorption states rickets is liable to develop after treatment has been started because it is a disease of growing bones. Vitamin D supplements should therefore be given.

Rickets may complicate renal disease under two quite different circumstances both of which are rare. *Glomerular* renal rickets may complicate chronic renal failure mainly because of the failure of the normal conversion in the kidney of 25-hydroxycholecalciferol to the active 1,25-dihydroxycholecalciferol. *Tubular* renal rickets results from a failure of normal tubular reabsorption of phosphate and may be a feature of many inborn errors of tubular function including vitamin-D resistant rickets and cystinosis. The rickets sometimes seen in children taking long-term anticonvulsants (especially phenytoin or barbiturates) is thought to be of renal origin.

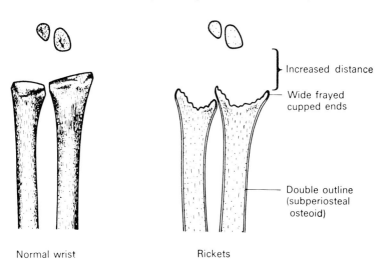

Normal wrist

Rickets

Increased distance

Wide frayed cupped ends

Double outline (subperiosteal osteoid)

Fig. 15. X-ray features of rickets.

The prevention of nutritional rickets can be assured by a daily vitamin D intake of 400 i.u. throughout infancy and early childhood. All baby milk foods and most cereals have vitamin D added. Infants are therefore likely to obtain sufficient from their diet, but pre-term babies should be given drops of vitamin concentrate for 6 months. Cod liver oil, although traditional, is probably the most unpleasant way to administer vitamin D and is no longer issued as a welfare food in Britain. The liability of Asian immigrant children to develop rickets is due more to nutritional deficiencies than to excess phytic acid. The treatment of established cases requires the education of the mother regarding the diet, and supplementary vitamin D, 5000 i.u. daily, until X-rays show healing. Excessive doses are dangerous. Renal rickets is more difficult to treat and requires careful and continuous metabolic control.

Scurvy

Scurvy is now a very rare disease amongst children in Britain. It is also rare in countries where malnutrition is prevalent because fruit is usually plentiful. In infancy the recommended vitamin C intake is 15 mg daily, although scurvy will probably not develop on half this amount. The predominant symptom of scurvy is haemorrhage, which may occur into the gums, the skin or subperiosteally. The last will cause severe limb pain so thay the child does not move the leg ('pseudo-paralysis') and screams at the approach of anyone who might touch it. X-rays show changes at the bone ends readily distinguished from those or rickets, with periosteal elevation and, later, calcification of subperiosteal haemorrhages. There is a rapid response to vitamin C.

SEXUAL DEVELOPMENT

Human sexual development is concentrated into two relatively brief periods of time. Primary sexual differentiation takes place from the 6th week of embryonic life. The gonad, which is undifferentiated up to this time, develops into a testicle in the presence of a Y chromosome or into an ovary in the presence of two X chromosomes.

The gonad then produces fetal hormones which influence the development of the Wolffian and Mullerian systems (gonaducts) along appropriate lines. The external genitalia develop a female pattern unless there are fetal androgens to masculinize them (Fig. 16).

Secondary sex characteristics develop at puberty in response to pituitary gonadotrophins. The trigger which releases these hormones is still unknown. The age of onset of puberty is very variable, being influenced by

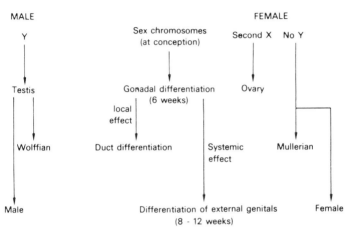

Fig. 16. Normal sex differentiation.

racial, hereditary and nutritional factors. In Britain today breast development begins at 11 years on average, pubic hair a little later and menstruation at 13, but ranging from 9 to 17 years: boys mature a little later. In both sexes, puberty is accompanied by an impressive growth spurt. Breast development in girls and growth of the testes and penis in boys are usually the first signs of puberty. Early breast development may be asymmetrical. Gonadal hormones are chiefly responsible for these changes, but adrenal androgens play a part (Fig. 17). The progress of puberty may be recorded in relation to the stages of pubic hair and breast development described by Tanner (Figs. 18a and b). Epiphyseal fusion, with cessation of growth, marks the end of puberty.

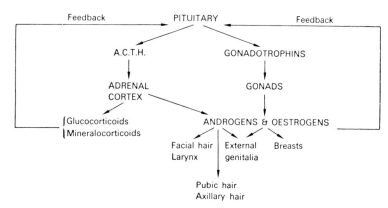

Fig. 17. Endocrine control of sex.

Intersex

The term is used to describe conditions in which the external genitalia at birth are not clearly appropriate to one sex or the other but show features of both. Some affected infants are masculinized genetic females; others are incompletely masculinized genetic males. The diagnostic problem is extremely urgent, partly because the most common underlying disorder is a dangerous one— the adrenogenital syndrome (p. 246)—and partly because prolonged uncertainty about the true sex is intolerable for the parents. Equally, much harm may be done if the wrong sex is assigned; later reversal may be traumatic. The 'right' sex is determined more by anatomy (functional possibilities) than by genetics.

Apart from the adrenogenital syndrome, causes of intersex are rare. Some progestational drugs given in pregnancy to discourage abortion may masculinize a female fetus. True hermaphrodites (with ovarian *and* testicular tissue) may have indeterminate genitalia. Investigation of intersex begins with a buccal smear, karyotyping and appropriate steroid chemistry.

Testicular feminization syndrome

In this rare but interesting condition there is a metabolic block in the activation of androgens in the tissues.

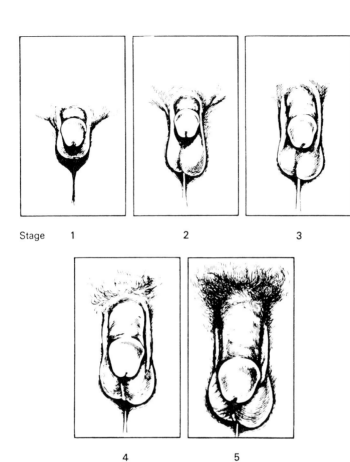

Stage   1   2   3

4   5

Fig. 18a. Stages of genital development:
1   Pre-adolescent
2   Enlargement of scrotum and testes
3   Lenthening of penis
4   Increase in breadth of penis and development of glans. Testes continue to enlarge. Scrotum darkens.
5   Adult. By this time pubic hair has spread to medial surface of thighs.

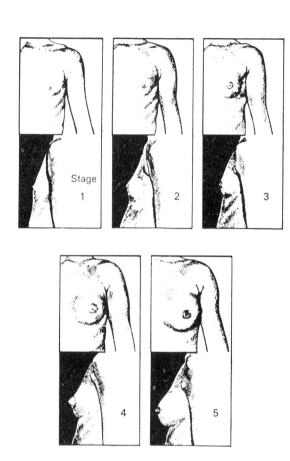

Fig. 18b. Stages of breast development:
1 Pre-adolescent: elevation of papilla only
2 Breast bud stage
3 Further enlargement of breast and areola
4 Projection of areola and papilla above level of breast
5 Mature stage, areola has recessed, papilla projects.

Affected individuals are genetic males with testicles, but the external genitalia are of a female pattern. Sometimes testes are palpable in the labia majora, or may be found at the time of operation for inguinal hernia. In some patients normal female secondary sexual characteristics develop at puberty if the testes are left in situ, but orchidectomy is advised later because of a definite risk of malignant change. The condition is due to a recessive gene and there is therefore a recurrence risk of 25% amongst siblings.

Late and early puberty

Children (especially boys) and their parents frequently seek advice about 'late' puberty. The vast majority are perfectly normal: they need reassurance and patience. Exceptionally there is pituitary or gonadal insufficiency.

Much less often the doctor is consulted about early (precocious) puberty. True precocious puberty includes spermatogenesis or oogenesis, and is rare. It results from **premature secretion of gonadotrophins.** Slightly less rare is precocious pseudopuberty, in which secondary sexual characteristics develop abnormally early, but there is no growth of the gonads and no gametogenesis. The isolated precocious development of breasts (mammarche or thelarche), periods (menarche) or pubic hair (pubarche or adrenarche) is commoner. Precocious puberty occurs more frequently in girls than in boys, and in the majority of instances the cause is unknown. A wide variety of intracranial disturbances, including tumours, hydrocephalus, meningitis and encephalitis, may lead to pubertal changes. Tumours arising in the adrenals or gonads may also cause precocious pseudo-puberty. Boys with the adrenogenital syndrome will develop precocious pseudo-puberty if left untreated. In the McCune–Albright syndrome precocious puberty is associated with tall stature, pigmented naevi and polyostotic fibrous dysplasia of bone. Each case requires careful examination and investigation.

Gynaecomastia in adolescent boys is almost always physiological and self-limiting. This does not prevent it being a considerable social embarrassment. Mastectomy may be justified if big breasts cause demoralisation.

Sex chromosome anomalies

These usually result from non-disjunction of sex chromosomes during gametogenesis in one or other parent. They disturb the development of the gonad much more than they influence the external genitalia and therefore rarely present before puberty except in the case of Turner's syndrome. Most children with abnormal sex chromosomes have normal external genitalia: most children with abnormal genitals (p. 62) have normal sex chromosomes.

The features of *Turner's syndrome*, which is usually associated with a single X chromosome, are short stature, webbed neck (pterygium colli), broad chest with wide-spaced nipples, and increased carrying angle at the elbows (cubitus valgus) (Fig. 19). Pigmented naevi are common. In some cases there is coarctation of the aorta. In many cases there is lymphoedema of the legs from birth, and this may be the first diagnostic pointer. Secondary sexual characteristics do not appear. The uterus and vagina may be small and the gonads are

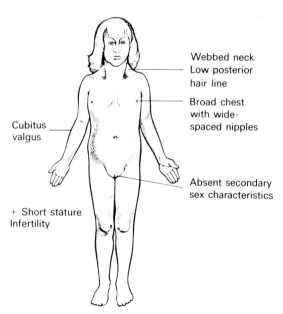

Webbed neck
Low posterior
hair line

Broad chest
with wide-
spaced nipples

Cubitus
valgus

Absent secondary
sex characteristics

+ Short stature
Infertility

Fig. 19. Turner's syndrome.

represented by rudimentary streaks in the edge of the broad ligament. Breast development and menstrual periods may be induced by hormone therapy, but affected individuals remain infertile and short.

In children suspected of sex chromosome anomalies a buccal smear should first be examined for chromatin bodies (Barr bodies) beneath the nuclear membrane. The number of bodies per cell is usually one less than the number of X chromosomes. The normal female (XX) has one: the normal male (XY) and the patients with Turner's syndrome (XO) have none. If the buccal smear is abnormal, the diagnosis should be confirmed by chromosome studies.

THE GENITALIA

Undescended testicles

The testicles normally descend into the scrotum about the 36th week of gestation and are therefore usually fully descended in the newborn full-term infant. Spontaneous descent may occur later, but the older the child the less likely is this to happen. If a testis remains undescended until after puberty it will not mature properly and will be sterile. 'Undescended' testicles are often incompletely descended and are palpable in the inguinal canal. If such a testis cannot be persuaded into the scrotum, or if the testis cannot be felt at all, orchidopexy is advised not later than 6 years of age.

Incompletely descended testes need to be distinguished from retractile testes and ectopic testes. Retractile testes are very common and normal. An active cremaster muscle will withdraw the testis into the inguinal canal or higher, especially if the doctor has cold hands. Ectopic testes are rare and may be located in the superficial inguinal pouch, near the femoral ring, or in the perineum.

Hydrocoele

At birth it is quite common to find fluid in the scrotal sac. It almost always clears up without treatment. In older infants and children there may be a tense hydrocoele on one or both sides. It does not cause symptoms but is often associated with inguinal hernia. Surgery is therefore advised.

Circumcision

The foreskin is normally adherent to the glans in the early months of life and sometimes for as long as 3 or 4 years. In infancy, therefore, the foreskin can only be retracted by breaking down the adhesions, a procedure which is unnecessary for the baby and distressing for the parents. A non-retractile prepuce in early life is therefore not an indication for circumcision. If the preputial orifice is small enough to obstruct urine flow (phimosis), circumcision is indicated. Paraphimosis is usually treated by an emergency dorsal slit followed later by circumcision.

Posthitis (inflammation of the foreskin) is common in baby boys while they are still in nappies. It requires treating as for nappy rash and is a contra-indication to circumcision because of the risk of a meatal ulcer. If normal separation of the foreskin from the glans does not occur by about the third year of life, or if the foreskin cannot be retracted in order to clean underneath then balanitis (inflammation of the glans) may occur and may be an indication for circumcision.

Hypospadias is a contra-indication to circumcision because the foreskin is used by the surgeon to fashion an anterior urethra.

Adherent labia minora

Sometimes firm adhesions develop between opposing surfaces of the labia minora (Fig. 20), probably as a consequence of poor personal hygiene. Urine is passed normally, but the appearance may suggest that there is no vaginal orifice. The labia may be separated with a probe or repeated application of oestrogen cream.

When having their perineum examined young girls are likely to be happiest if lying supine on their mother's lap or on a couch with their legs up in the lithotomy position. They can see what the examiner is up to. The labia are gently pulled apart to check that they are not adherent and the vulva is inspected. Vaginal examination is a little more difficult. If the child crouches forward in the

Fig. 20. Adherent labia. The labia are adherent throughout most of their length but a small orifice remains through which urine is passed (N.B. the orifice is not the vagina).

prone position with the chest well down, the knees slightly apart, and the bottom stuck in the air this tends to open the vagina and reasonable inspection can be done using a torch and without the need to put anything in the vagina.

Vaginal discharge

Soreness and irritation of the vulva in girls is nearly always due to a lack of personal hygiene. Micturition may be painful. A mucoid vaginal discharge, recognized by the mother from staining of the knickers, results from the normal secretion of mucus in a rather larger amount than usual. Careful daily washing and drying of the perineum will relieve both conditions.

A purulent vaginal discharge in childhood is less common. Pus should be cultured and examined for Trichomonas. The possibility of an underlying foreign body should be borne in mind. *Vaginal bleeding* due to oestrogen withdrawal may occur in infants about a week old. Bleeding in older girls is rare and may be due to normal or precocious menarche, foreign body or tumour. Internal examination under anaesthesia may be needed.

The causes of vaginal discharge are summarized below:

White mucoid (leukorrhoea):
(a) in neonate, normal,
(b) at puberty, normal.
Offensive yellow (vulvovaginitis):
(a) age 2–5, associated with poor hygiene,
(b) infection or foreign body.
Bloody (vaginal bleeding):
(a) in neonate may be normal,
(b) foreign body,
(c) tumour,
(d) menarche.

Further reading

Tanner J. M. *Foetus into Man*. Open Books.
Buckler J. M. H. *A Reference Manual of Growth and Development*. Blackwell Scientific Publications.
Falkner F. and Tanner J. M. *Human Growth*. Ballière, Tindall.

Chapter 5

Developmental Assessment

Developmental testing is a routine part of the examination of any child, especially infants and young children. The purpose is to identify developmental delay early so that, if possible, the cause may be corrected and appropriate help organised for the child and the family. There are standards for the age at which normal children achieve particular skills (Appendix 7). Few people can remember all these 'milestones', but everyone needs to learn a few. The skills can be divided into four main categories:

1   Posture and movement;
2   Vision and manipulation;
3   Hearing and speech;
4   Social behaviour.

The starting point is to learn these four categories and then to learn one or two skills which fit into each category. There are two parts to a developmental assessment.

(a) *The history.* The mother should be encouraged to give a careful account of the child's present skills, ensuring that each of the four main categories is covered. If there are older siblings it is helpful to enquire how the child's skills compare with those of the sibling at that age. Enquire about school performance if the child is at school for he is unlikely to have a significant developmental problem if he is coping well in a normal class of children of similar age. Secondly, try to obtain information about the dates of the early milestones. Some mothers recall them well, and others not at all. If an experienced mother says 'he was very quick' it may not be necessary to obtain exact details of past achievements.

(b) *Play with the child*—in the presence of the mother so as to encourage the child to show certain skills.

Try to define the limit of achievement by noting both the skills the child *has* and those he has *not*. The Denver Developmental Screening Test charts are useful for recording information, and for practising developmental assessment. The following simple tests require equipment that is available in any surgery or clinic, and require no special expertise on the part of the examiner. The ages given are the *average* ages at which the skill is seen.

1 Posture and movement

Pulled to sitting, the head comes up in a line with the trunk by 3 months, and is then held steady as the child is supported sitting.

Sitting—a child sits unsupported for 1 minute at 7 months, and for 10 minutes at 9 months.

Walking—at 6 months a child starts to take weight on his legs, at 9 months he bounces or stamps when supported and at 13 months he takes 10 steps unsupported.

2 Vision and manipulation (hand–eye coordination)

Visual attention. At 8 weeks a baby observes with a convergent gaze a dangling toy or bright object held 9–12 inches from his face, and moves his head and neck in order to follow it. A true squint (as distinct from a pseudo-squint as seen with epicanthic folds) is always abnormal and requires referral to a specialist (see p. 79).

From 2 months a baby prefers to watch a face rather than anything else, but more detailed testing is possible with care and special equipment. The Stycar testing kit includes:

(a) a series of white balls of different sizes which are rolled across the floor in front of the baby. At 6–9 months a baby will watch a ball as small as $\frac{1}{4}$ inch diameter at a distance of 10 feet.

(b) two sets of miniature dolls-house type toys and cutlery. The toddler has one set and points to the item which is the same as that held by the tester 10 feet away.

(c) letter matching cards which can be used at 3–6 years, even though the child has not yet learnt letters. The child points to one of the five letters on his card which is the same as a single letter displayed by the tester 10 feet away.

Grasp. A wooden tongue depressor or spatula is held before the infant. At 6 months he approaches it with the ulnar border of the hand and then takes it in a clumsy palmar grasp. At 9 months he approaches it with the radial border and takes it in a scissor grasp between the sides of thumb and index finger before transferring it to the other hand and putting it in his mouth. At 12 months he approaches it with the index finger and picks it up precisely between the ends of the thumb and index finger in a pincer grasp (Fig. 21).

6 months   9 months   12 months

Fig. 21. Palmar grasp at 6 months, scissor grasp at 9 months, pincer grasp at 12 months.

Copying. A child will copy with a pencil the following shapes

| or — at 2 years	□ at 5 years
○ at 3 years	△ at 6 years
+ at 4 years	◇ at 7 years

Building and copying with blocks. Small wooden 1 inch cubes are best. The child will copy:

at 1½ years a tower of
3 cubes   at 3 a 'bridge' is copied

at 2 years a tower of   at 3½ a 'train'
6–8 cubes

                                   at 4 'steps'

3 Hearing and speech

Localization of sounds. The baby is sat on mother's knee facing forward. A variety of soft sounds are made lateral to either ear and out of the line of vision. Rustling soft tissue or toilet paper provides a high frequency sound; a spoon gently scraped round a cup, or a spin rattle are other suitable sounds. Provided the baby has reasonable vision (and hearing) he will turn to locate the source. At 7 months the baby turns to sounds $1\frac{1}{2}$ feet from either ear. At 9 months he turns promptly to sounds 3 feet away, even if they are situated diagonally (Fig. 22), and at 12 months localizes sounds made vertically above his head. The optimal age at which to test an infant's hearing is 9 months, before insatiable curiosity for new sounds gives way to the contemptuous boredom with which a sophisticated 15-month-old treats the tests.

Speech. At 9 months there is varied and tuneful babbling. From 1 year single word *labels* are used for familiar objects and people—'Mum', 'Dog'. He will look

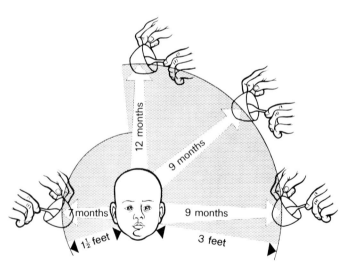

Fig. 22. Hearing responses in first year. At seven months the sound should be made $1\frac{1}{2}$ ft lateral to the ear. From 9 months the sound can be made 3 ft lateral to the ear.

towards a named object e.g. 'where's the ball?' At 2 years
words are joined to convey *ideas*—'Dadad gone' and will
follow simple instructions e.g. 'put the spoon in the cup'.
At 3 sentences are used to describe present and past
happenings. Throughout this period the child's understanding of language is far ahead of his ability to utter it.

4   Social behaviour

Smiling. In response to mother's face smiling is seen at
4–8 weeks.

   Reacting to strangers. Up to 9 months most babies will
be happily handled by anyone, from 9 months they begin
to cry or fret if handled by a stranger.

   Feeding. At 9 months lumpy food is properly chewed. At
18 months the child cooperates with feeding, and drinks
from an ordinary cup using two hands. At 3 years he can
feed himself efficiently with a spoon and fork.

LIMITATIONS OF DEVELOPMENTAL ASSESSMENT

Technique

As with any examination the expert will always get the
most reliable information, but anyone who is willing to
listen to the mother and observe the child can get some
useful information about each of the four main fields of
development. If the mother's account differs greatly from
what is observed, it may be that the child is having an 'off
day', in which case observing on another occasion will be
more reliable.

Range of normal

The age at which a normal child achieves a particular
physical or developmental goal is extremely variable:
50% of children can walk 10 steps unaided at 13 months,
but a few can do this at 8 months, and others not until 18
months. It is kinder to talk to parents of the 'usual' age for
developing a skill rather than the 'normal', since abnormal implies a fault. Quite commonly one field of activity

appears delayed in a normal child, but it is rare for all four fields of development to be delayed if the child is normal.

Milestones are stepping stones

Parents tend to think of certain developmental skills as essential milestones. It is truer to regard them as stepping stones. In general one cannot reach a particular stepping stone without using the previous ones—and a child does not run until he can walk or walk until he can stand. But different people may use different stepping stones, and occasionally miss one out. Most children crawl before they stand, but some shuffle on their bottoms, never crawl, yet stand and walk normally in the end. Bottom shuffling is a typical example of the sort of variation in development that can cause parents much unnecessary worry, particularly as bottom shufflers tend to walk later than other children.

Using stepping stones we may go in sudden bounds rather than at an even rate—children often develop that way, appearing static for a few weeks then suddenly mastering a new skill. If the next stepping stone is a particularly hard one all the child's energy may appear to be devoted to just one of the four fields of development, whilst the other three seem static; posture and movement skills may advance rapidly about the age of 1 year as walking is mastered, whilst hearing and speech development appear static.

The first 6 months

This is the most difficult time to assess the baby, because it is not until about 6 months that many of the easier developmental tests can be used. Therefore, developmental testing before the age of 6 months is less reliable than at any other time.

THE SLOW CHILD

'He is slow at walking', 'She is late at talking'. Such worries are common reasons for parents consulting the doctor. Usually the parents are correct that their child is later than usual at achieving a particular skill. The cause will be found in one of the following six categories.

1 motor fault;
2 sensory fault;
3 learning fault (low intelligence);
4 psychological fault;
5 social deprivation;
6 late normal.

In general practice the commonest reason is 'late normal', that is a normal child who happens to be at one end of the age range at which that skill is achieved. But one cannot reassure the parents that the reason is 'late normal' until a history and examination have excluded the other reasons. For instance if the child of 2 does not say words check the six categories:

1 motor—is he unable to use the palate and larynx because of cerebral palsy?
2 sensory—is he deaf?
3 learning—is he of low intelligence, i.e. mentally handicapped?
4 psychological—is there severe psychological illnesses (autism may present as slowness in talking)?
5 social—has the child been exposed to speech, or been left all day in the care of a baby minder who speaks a different language from the parents?
6 late normal?

Language disorders

Medical advice may be sought about children who do not talk, or about those who talk but have defective speech. The problems involve three main areas:

1 Language skills:
    (a) understanding speech,
    (b) speaking.
2 Fluency e.g. stammer.
3 Voice and resonance, e.g. as a result of hypernasality or cleft palate.

Some children have a sizable vocabulary before their first birthday while others say little until 3 or 4 years of age. If talking is delayed it is important to search for a reason as described above. In most instances there are no specific barriers to speech and it will develop naturally, but early assessment is important so that appropriate help can be given early. It is important to explain to parents how they can help their child to talk well. Speech is encouraged by the child being spoken to, and read to, and by mixing with other talkative children.

Poor fluency is common in young children and can be considered normal in toddlers. But if it persists it renders the child unintelligible and he becomes frustrated by the apparent stupidity of others. Stuttering (stammering) usually starts between 2 and 4 years of age. Stutter rarely begins after the age of 7. It is much commoner in boys and most lose their stutter spontaneously. On the whole it seems that the less attention that is drawn to the stutter the better. However, for more severe and persistent problems speech therapy is extremely helpful and prevents it from becoming permanent.

There is a strong link between language delay and later educational difficulties. Therefore, the child with such delay should be assessed as early and expertly as possible.

School difficulties

If a healthy child of normal intelligence and good vision and hearing has educational difficulties, an emotional problem will often be found. There may be unhappiness at home, or at school (from bullying or fear of a teacher), or parental over-expectation or under-expectation. Conversely, emotional problems may be the result of learning problems. A report from the school is an important part of the assessment of the school child.

When a child's reading ability is more than 2 years behind that which is expected for his *age*, he is said to have reading backwardness. This is a common condition of boys and girls, particularly in those from social classes IV and V, and in children with an overt neurological disorder or a mild neurodevelopmental fault. A smaller group of children are said to have *specific reading retardation*: their reading age is more than 2 years behind their *mental age* (as measured by IQ testing). They are much worse at reading, speech and language than at other skills, and are particularly recalcitrant to treatment. This is commoner in boys and occurs in all social classes. It is not associated with neurological abnormalities. Some of these children are sometimes referred to as suffering from '*dyslexia*', but the term is falling out of favour because of early inaccurate descriptions of it. All types of reading problems are commoner in large families, and all children with them need skilled assessment and help. Educational and clinical psychologists have an important role in the evaluation and management of children who have difficulty in acquiring specific skills.

Severe *clumsiness* is another important cause of school difficulties. Apart from difficulty with dressing or physical activities, some clumsy children may have great difficulty with writing and drawing. They may be considered wrongly to be stupid or lazy. Some authorities consider very clumsy children to be suffering from 'minimal brain damage' (p. 102). Others affix imposing labels such as 'developmental dystaxia'; whatever the label, once the problem is recognised the children can be taught to overcome many of the problems.

SQUINT (STRABISMUS)

Nearly 1 in 15 children have a squint when they commence school. The incidence is even greater in children with brain damage or mental handicap.

Babies sometimes falsely give the impression of having a squint because of a low nasal bridge, epicanthic folds, or wide-spaced eyes (hypertelorism). This is a pseudo-squint and unimportant. But a true squint is always abnormal.

To detect a squint the child is encouraged to look at an interesting object held in different directions. Full eye movements are limited. With a *paralytic squint* the deviation of one eye becomes more marked in a particular direction of gaze, whereas a child with the commoner *concomitant squint* has the same deviation in all directions. It is useful to observe the reflection of a torchlight in the cornea. The child observes the light as it is moved in different directions. A child with a squint shows the reflection in the centre of one pupil, but eccentric in the other. For all children except small babies it is usually possible to use the cover test. The child looks at an object, the examiner covers one eye with a hand or a book and observes the uncovered eye carefully. If the eye has a squint (and has not yet developed amblyopia) it will move to fix on the object when the good eye is covered. A normal eye does not move when the defective eye is covered. For this test it is important that the object is held within 30 cm of the child's face.

Any child with a squint should be referred to an eye specialist. He excludes the rare but serious causes for a squint which include cataract, glaucoma, retinal disease and retinoblastoma, and then organises a plan of management. An untreated squint may cause the child to adopt an unusual tilt of the head or other posture to improve binocular vision in certain directions. More seriously, a young child suppresses the information from the defective eye in order to avoid blurred images and double vision. Unused the eye becomes 'lazy' and can develop permanent *amblyopia* (diminished acuity of central vision). Treatment before the age of 6 should always prevent this. After the age of 10 a 'lazy eye' is likely to remain useless for life. A common treatment for young children, which is as unpopular with them as it is with their parents, is for the good eye to be occluded with a patch in order to force the child to use the lazy eye. This is often done for a period of several months before spectacles or other treatment is offered. With patience and determination children over the age of $1\frac{1}{2}$ years can be persuaded to keep patches or spectacles on most of the time.

For many young children with a squint resulting from poor visual acuity, early use of spectacles is sufficient treatment in itself. Severe squints, particularly if paralytic, may require surgery—if only for cosmetic reasons. After operation orthoptic exercises may be organised to encourage the child to stimulate binocular function.

BLINDNESS

Severe visual impairment is a terrible handicap at any age. When it is congenital, or even when its origin is in the pre-school years, it presents a serious threat to satisfactory development and education.

Local authorities keep a register of children with severe visual problems so that the families can be helped and suitable education planned. Experienced home advisors from either the local authority or the RNIB (Royal

National Institute for the Blind—a charitable organisation) visit the family to provide continuing advice and support. They provide practical advice e.g. 'wear noisy shoes and give a running commentary about all your household activities so that he can understand and learn about the things he hears, sometimes smells and feels, but never sees'. Severe visual impairment requires formal education by methods not involving the use of sight; the specialist schools for the blind teach braille. For children with sufficient sight to use educational material involving large print and type, there are residential schools for the 'partially sighted'. Both types of school are few in number, and the child is almost certain to be resident in one some distance from home.

Further reading

Sheridan, Mary *The Developmental Progress of Infants and Young Children*. Her Majesty's Stationery Office.

Egan D., Illingworth R.S. and MacKeith R.C. *Developmental Screening 0–5*. Clinics in Developmental Medicine No. 20. W. Heinemann Medical Books.

Illingworth R. S. *The Development of the Infant and Young Child*. Churchill-Livingstone.

Denver Developmental Screening Test. *J. Paediatrics* 1967; **71:** 185. (The charts are available from The Test Agency, Counswood House, North Dean, High Wycombe, Buckinghamshire.)

Chapter 6

The Nervous System

Brain growth occurs early in life, and is largely complete by the age of 2 years. Myelination is mainly complete by the age of 3, but both myelination and arborisation (the establishment of dendritic connections) continue to a small extent up to the age of 5. The brain is particularly vulnerable during this early period. Malnutrition and other adverse factors in utero or in early life may limit brain growth and affect brain function in a manner that does not occur in later life. Thus prolonged deficiency of thyroid hormone in the newborn leads to irreversible mental handicap, whereas in the older child or adult lethargic behaviour is reversed by treatment.

Conventional examination of the nervous system has to be modified considerably for children, particularly young children. As is the case with so many childhood examinations careful *inspection* is of great importance. A few minutes spent sitting near the young child, observing him closely, may yield as much information as the rest of the examination. In the baby, the doctor is observing posture and movement, and looking for abnormal postures, for the level of spontaneous activity, for abnormal movements and asymmetry of movement. The toddler is best watched at play, particular interest being paid to gait and manipulative skills; ataxia, tremors, abnormal hand postures or weakness of a limb are easily seen. Much more information is gleaned from detailed observation of the contented infant or toddler at play, than from the unhappy young child who is thrust supine on a bed and subjected to a conventional adult type of neurological examination, even though certain aspects of such an examination are helpful in children as well as

adults.

Assessment of *tone* is particularly useful, and it is worth handling many young children to become familiar with normal tone. In infants the head should be facing directly forwards; if it is facing to one side the asymmetric neck reflex (p. 84) may cause disparity in tone between the two sides. Tendon reflexes are easier to elicit in a child's legs than arms. Most children are more relaxed when sitting than lying and the leg tendon reflexes will be elicited more easily when the child's legs are dangling down from the chair, with the examiner lightly grasping the child's foot for the ankle jerk or the child's leg for the knee jerk. If no response is obtained the degree of flexion of the foot or knee should be altered slightly and the test repeated. In young children the plantar response can be obtained by holding the foot steady and scratching along the lateral side of the sole from the toes towards the heel; this avoids eliciting the primitive plantar flexion grasp response which is present in infants and in children with cerebral damage (see below). The true plantar response is extensor in infants and may not become flexor until 2–3 years of age.

The fundi may be difficult to see in uncooperative children. Older children will keep their eyes still whilst being examined if given an interesting object on which to fix (provided the doctor keeps his head out of the way!). Young children struggle against having their eyelids held apart, and the doctor is more likely to see the fundi of a 3-year-old if he keeps his hands off the child's face altogether. Infants will often be still and looking up with wide open eyes during a feed. Otherwise, firm assisting hands may be needed to examine the fundi of struggling infants and toddlers and it may be necessary both to sedate the infant beforehand and to apply a mydriatic such as tropicamide in order to see the fundi satisfactorily.

The neurological examination of infants has to include some additional items:

The head

The maximum occipito-frontal *head circumference* is noted and compared with the normal (Appendix 1). The fontanelles are palpated. The *anterior fontanelle* is variable in shape and size but has an average diameter of 2 cm during the first 9 months. It closes between 12 and 18 months. It should feel soft. A bulging or tense fontanelle is common in crying infants; in a quiet infant it is a sign of raised intracranial pressure.

Primitive reflexes

These reflexes are present in early life but disappear as myelination is completed and cortical control develops. They vary in intensity during the early months, start to go from 3 months and should be gone by 6 months. A strongly positive primitive reflex after 6 months indicates cerebral damage. Examples of such primitive reflexes are:
(a) The Moro reflex which occurs in response to many stimuli. One method of eliciting it is to hold the baby supine with the head supported in one hand. When the head is allowed to drop 2 inches onto the other hand, there is sudden extension and abduction of the upper limbs, with opening of the hands, followed by flexion to the midline. The movement should be symmetrical.
(b) The plantar and palmar grasp reflexes, in which flexion of the fingers or toes occurs in response to a finger being pressed on the palm or sole respectively, and are released by pressure along the extensor surface of the fingers or toes.
(c) Asymmetrical tonic neck reflex. As the infant turns his head to the side, the limbs on the chin side extend and those on the occipital side flex (Fig. 27, p. 101). This reflex is maximal at the age of 3 months.

There is sometimes confusion between the neurological examination of infants and developmental assessment. Both are equally important, but though they are linked with each other it is best to consider and record them separately. Developmental assessment (Chapter 5) is primarily concerned with the achievement of learned skills. Neurological examination is primarily concerned with normal and abnormal anatomy and physiology of the nervous system. Primitive reflexes, for instance, are involuntary reactions to stimuli (some people call them 'infantile automatisms'), and even though they develop and change during the early months they are best included in the neurological examination rather than the developmental assessment.

SEIZURES

A seizure is the result of an abnormal paroxysmal discharge of cerebral neurones. Seizures are called different names by different people—'seizure', 'fit', 'convulsion', 'blackout', 'turn' or 'attack', the last three being used more by patients than by doctors.

People who have more than one non-febrile convulsion are said to have epilepsy. They have a tendency to recurrent seizures. Electroencephalography (EEG) is usually abnormal immediately after a fit, but may be normal 2 weeks later. However, 60% of people who have epilepsy have consistently abnormal EEGs between fits.

Fits are common in childhood: 6% of children have had a fit by the age of 11 years. The pattern and prognosis varies with age (Fig. 23).

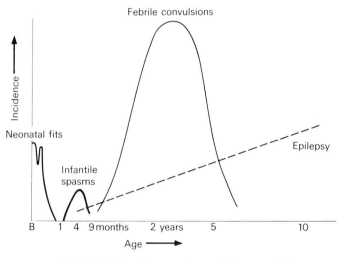

Fig. 23. The incidence and type of seizure at different ages.

1   Neonatal seizures

Seizures are common in the first month as a result of birth injury, metabolic and infective causes or developmental abnormalities (further details are given on p. 42).

2 Infantile spasms

Infantile spasms are a rare and serious form of seizure characteristically commencing between the ages of 1 month and 6 months. The infant doubles up, flexing at the waist and neck, and flinging the arms forward—a 'salaam' spasm; less commonly it is an extensor spasm. Associated mental subnormality is common. The EEG usually shows a characteristically disorganised picture—hypsarrhythmia. Corticosteroids may suppress the fits. The final outcome is related to the cause, which may be a metabolic fault, a congenital structural abnormality of the brain or various other forms of brain damage. Quite often no cause is found.

3 Febrile convulsions

Four per cent of pre-school children have a seizure. By far the commonest is a febrile convulsion, which is defined as a seizure occurring between 3 months and 5 years of age associated with fever but without evidence of intra-cranial infection or defined cause. Although they may be recurrent they should be distinguished from epilepsy (which is characterised by recurrent non-febrile seizures). A family history of seizures is often present.

The seizures are generalised with clonic movements usually lasting less than 10 minutes. They are precipitated by a febrile illness rather than by fever itself and tend to occur at the start of the illness. Upper respiratory tract infections are the commonest association. The CNS is normal and there are no neurological signs once the seizure has ceased. Half the children will have further febrile convulsions with future illnesses, but less than 15% have seizures after the age of 6. Prolonged, focal or frequent seizures, or an EEG which is abnormal more than 2 weeks after the seizure make the likelihood of seizures in later life, that is epilepsy, greater.

Seizures are frightening to the family and it is common for the parents to think their child is dying. In addition to reassurance immediate therapy consists of:

(a) Laying the child semi-prone with the neck slightly extended so that secretions drain out of the mouth and do not obstruct the airway.

(b) Cooling the child. Antipyretics such as aspirin are helpful. Excess clothing or bedclothes should be removed. Occasionally sponging with tepid water (which does not cause skin vasoconstriction) is needed.

(c) Antibiotics, if an infection such as otitis media is present.

(d) Anticonvulsants, which are continued while the child is febrile.

The main problem for the doctor is in deciding whether to admit the child to hospital. If there is any suspicion of meningitis admission is necessary for lumbar puncture. If there is clear evidence of an associated infection home treatment is reasonable, particularly if there is a previous history of febrile convulsions.

Long-term management consists of explaining to the parents the relatively benign nature of febrile seizures and teaching them how to recognise and manage future seizures, use antipyretic agents safely and effectively, first aid for a seizure, and when and how to seek emergency assistance. Long-term prophylactic anticonvulsant therapy is sometimes used for selected children with recurrent febrile convulsions.

4 Epilepsy

Idiopathic epilepsy is the usual reason for seizures in schoolchildren. Approximately 1 in 200 schoolchildren are affected. The child is healthy and normal on examination, but has recurrent seizures which may be generalised or partial.

Generalised seizures

Grand mal

These are major convulsions which classically have a tonic phase, clonic phase, then a period of unconsciousness followed by confusion and/or drowsiness for up to an hour (quite commonly the child will sleep after the seizure). There may be some preceding aura. In some children photic stimulation is a provocative factor; if it is associated with watching the television it may be called *television epilepsy*. Such children are advised to sit at least 10 feet away from the television, avoid adjusting the set, look away if there is flickering or cover one eye if feeling odd. Therapy for grand mal epilepsy includes phenytoin, phenobarbitone, sodium valproate and carbamazepine.

Petit mal

This is a very brief absence of awareness lasting less than 5 seconds accompanied by eye blinking. The child does not fall down. It may be unrecognised until the child presents with school difficulties because of 'day dreaming' or 'poor attention'.

Petit mal can be provoked by encouraging the child to hyperventilate. Petit mal is uncommon; the onset is always in childhood. The characteristic EEG is 3 per second spike and wave pattern. It is never caused by organic brain damage and the intelligence and behaviour of the child are normal. Sodium valproate or ethosuximide are the most effective drugs.

Partial seizures (focal epilepsy)

The seizure discharge is confined to a focus of neurones and does not become generalised. Sometimes the focus is at the site of previous cerebral damage (for example some children with temporal lobe epilepsy have acquired it as a result of anoxic damage to the temporal lobe during a prolonged convulsion). Carbamazepine is a particularly effective treatment. The most important types are:

Temporal lobe

Temporal lobe lesions are the cause of complex partial seizures (*psychomotor epilepsy*). They are a more common reason for minor fits than petit mal, and may present as motor, sensory or emotional phenomena singly or in combination. Any convulsive movements are less repetitive than Jacksonian seizures. The diagnosis is confirmed by EEG. The children, especially the boys, may have psychiatric and behaviour problems and, occasionally, impaired intelligence.

Jacksonian (minor motor seizures)

These are simple partial seizures which may occur without any disturbance of consciousness. The convulsive movement predominantly affects one area of the body only, though the clinical manifestations may 'march' to involve the corner of the mouth and the periocular muscles. Sometimes the seizure is followed by temporary paralysis or weakness of a limb (*Todds paralysis*). Jacksonian fits in children have a less serious prognosis than in adults.

General management of epilepsy

Although most seizures are idiopathic it is important to search for a primary cause from a careful history and examination, for fits can be caused by space-occupying lesions, meningitis, hypoglycaemia, hypertension, and many other causes. A rare but interesting group are children with neurocutaneous syndromes in which a skin lesion is associated with an intracranial lesion. Many of these are genetically determined and associated with mental handicap. It is customary to examine carefully the child's skin for the pathognomonic skin lesion:

Sturge–Weber: port wine stain (p. 201).

Neurofibromatosis: café-au-lait spots.

Tuberose sclerosis (epiloia): depigmented and pigmented areas, particularly on the trunk and, later on, papules over the nose and face (adenoma sebaceum).

The principles of anticonvulsant therapy are to use the lowest dose of the safest drug that suppresses fits and to continue the drug until at least 2 years after the last fit. Children metabolise anticonvulsant drugs faster than adults so that a single daily dose is less likely to be effective in childhood. An additional problem with phenobarbitone is that it causes hyperkinesis and behaviour problems in some children. Both phenytoin and phenobarbitone predispose to rickets, particularly in institutionalised children receiving a poor diet and little sunshine. The advent of modern anticonvulsant drugs has reduced greatly the number of children with intractable epilepsy who require treatment with a ketogenic diet, or with neurosurgery.

Most children with epilepsy attend normal school; only a tiny minority have such intractable epilepsy that special schooling is required. It is important that the teachers are informed so that they may recognise and deal with any seizure. Although the child should take part in most activities he may need extra supervision for swimming, and it may be wisest to prevent him from doing activities such as high diving, rope or rock climbing, and canoeing. Some doctors forbid cycling in traffic if the child has had a seizure in the previous 2 years, though seizures are uncommon during any concentrated activity.

Status epilepticus refers to the state in which a child convulses or has a series of convulsions for over 60 minutes without recovering consciousness in between. Apart from external injury, brain damage may result. Therefore all fits must be stopped fast. Intravenous diazepam is the drug of choice in hospital. At home intramuscular paraldehyde, into the lateral side of the thigh to avoid the sciatic nerve, is most effective. This is combined with securing an adequate airway, administering oxygen, protecting the child from injury and, over a longer period, maintaining fluid and electrolyte balance.

Conditions simulating epilepsy

Faints are uncommon below the age of 10, but are common in adolescent schoolgirls. In contrast to fits the girl remembers feeling dizzy beforehand, and is not sleepy afterwards. Pallor and sweating may accompany the faint.

Breath-holding attacks (see p. 128).

Benign paroxysmal vertigo usually starts in young school children. There may be brief recurrent attacks of dizziness, somtimes with sweating and vomiting, but no loss of consciousness. Nystagmus may be present.

Masturbatory episodes in infants and toddlers may mimic fits. The child may sit or lie with legs squeezed together, or rock to and fro. He may be flushed, breathless or may utter a shriek.

Acute infantile hemiplegia presents as a seizure, and is a rare but serious condition. A previously healthy young child has severe convulsions, often unilateral, becomes comatose and develops hemiplegia. Vascular causes are suspected, but rarely identified. Some people believe the hemiplegia is the result of anoxic damage from the prolonged fit. Recovery is slow and incomplete in that the child usually has a residual weakness of one side, intellectual impairment or epilepsy.

Night terrors (see p. 127).

MENINGITIS

This is essentially a childhood disease: 80% of all cases of meningitis occur in the first 5 years of life. Children aged 6–12 months are at greatest risk.

The early symptoms and signs may be non-specific, particularly in infants. Fever, vomiting, headache and irritability are usual; the older child may complain of neck-ache. Fits are common and increasing drowsiness precedes coma.

In infancy the main sign of meningitis is a bulging anterior fontanelle; head retraction is common but it is difficult to elicit neck stiffness in infants. Older children do have pronounced neck stiffness and this is best demonstrated by persuading the child to look down at an object, to press the examiner's finger against his chest with his chin, or to kiss his own knees. This is a more reliable method than the examiner forcefully flexing the child's head, which many children without meningitis resist.

Common viral causes of meningitis (aseptic meningitis) are mumps and echoviruses. Mumps meningitis often occurs in the absence of other manifestations of mumps and is especially common in boys. Poliomyelitis, once a common and serious form of aseptic meningitis, is hardly ever seen in countries which provide mass immunization against the disease. Bacterial causes of meningitis (purulent meningitis) are slightly less common than viral causes but more serious and more likely to cause brain injury. In neonates meningitis may be caused by a wide variety of different micro-organisms, *Escherichia coli* being the commonest. In childhood the three main pathogens are *Neisseria meningitidis* (gram-negative diplococcus), *Haemophilus influenzae* (gram-negative bacillus) and *Streptococcus pneumoniae* (gram-positive diplococcus).

91

Investigation

Prompt lumbar puncture is imperative. Papilloedema is not a contra-indication, provided only 1–2 ml of CSF are removed. Gram stain and differential cell count provide the most useful immediate information. Usually it is possible to differentiate an aseptic meningitis from a purulent meningitis from the CSF examination as shown in Table 6, provided the child has not received recent antibiotics.

Table 6. Characteristics of CSF

	Normal	Aseptic meningitis	Purulent meningitis
Appearance	Clear	Clear or hazy	Cloudy or purulent
Cells/mm^3	0–4	20–1000	1000–5000
Type	Lymphocytes	Lymphocytes	Polymorphs
Protein g/l	0·2–0·4	0·2–1·0	0·4–10
Glucose mmol/l	3–6	3–6	0·5–6

When the findings are equivocal it is usual to treat as if there is a bacterial pathogen. Tuberculous meningitis (p. 272) may present as a lymphocytic meningitis. Faeces, CSF and throat swabs can be cultured for viruses, and in all cases blood culture should be performed. The ESR may be of help in meningitis, for a value of over 50 makes a viral aetiology (aseptic meningitis) most improbable.

Treatment

Children with purulent meningitis are treated initially with intravenous antibiotics. Until the bacterium has been identified chloramphenicol and large doses of ampicillin may be used. This is combined with whatever supportive and symptomatic therapy may be needed—anticonvulsants, analgesics, or intravenous fluids for a collapsed child. Improvement should occur within 36 hours, and early treatment is usually associated with complete recovery. Slow recovery or relapse may be a sign of persisting infection or of a subdural effusion. Aspiration and drainage of the effusion is needed.

Outcome

Meningitis is a serious condition. Some children die and a proportion incur permanent brain damage resulting in deafness, mental handicap or cerebral palsy. These problems and secondary hydrocephalus are more likely in infants. Aseptic meningitis is treated symptomatically and has a lower incidence of complications. Recurrent meningitis is most rare, and should provoke a close search for a dermal sinus. This is a small pit found in the midline of the back which provides a portal through which micro-organisms reach the meninges. Immunological disorders may also present with recurrent meningitis.

Meningococcal septicaemia

This may occur with or without associated meningitis. It is a serious and frightening condition which is endemic in Britain. Small epidemics sometimes occur, though the infectivity within households is low. Pre-school children are most severely affected. The onset is abrupt and the course may be catastrophically fulminating with death occurring within 12 hours. The pathognomic sign is a purpuric rash, which may be sparse or so profuse that the lesions coalesce to form large ecchymoses. One mode of death is from peripheral circulatory failure associated with haemorrhage into the adrenal glands (*Waterhouse–Friederichsen syndrome*). An intravenous infusion should be set up on any child suspected of having menigococcal septicaemia; antibiotics are given intravenously, and the line can be used for plasma expanders or hydrocortisone in the event of collapse.

Encephalitis

Encephalitis is an illness in which cerebral symptoms (e.g. fits and drowsiness) or neurological signs are not accompanied by definite signs of meningitis. The CSF usually has raised protein and/or lymphocytes. The commonest form in childhood is acute disseminated encephalomyelitis associated with infection (also called meningo-encephalitis or post-infectious encephalitis). It is not caused by direct infective invasion of the brain, and usually occurs about a week after one of the common infectious fevers—measles, rubella, chicken pox or mumps. Most cases are mild, but occasionally severe and permanent brain damage ensues as a result of demyelination.

Meningism

This is the term given to the symptoms and signs, particularly the neck stiffness, that may be present at the time of an extracranial infection. It may be associated with otitis media, tonsilitis, cervical adenitis or pneumonia. Often a lumbar puncture has to be done to ensure that the CSF is normal and the child has not got meningitis.

HYDROCEPHALUS

Hydrocephalus arises from obstruction to the normal CSF circulation either as a result of congenital abnormality, e.g. aqueduct stenosis, or from post-natal causes such as meningitis, intracranial haemorrhage or tumour. It is commonly associated with spina bifida.

In congenital hydrocephalus the size of the head at birth varies from normal to such gross enlargement that the infant can only be delivered after destruction of the skull.

As the CSF accumulates under pressure the head enlarges rapidly, the skull sutures separate, the anterior fontanelle bulges and the scalp veins appear prominent. The eyes turn downward (setting sun sign). In the older child whose skull sutures are united, obstruction to CSF causes headache, vomiting and other symptoms of raised intracranial pressure. It is the rate of skull expansion rather than any single skull circumference measurement that has to be measured in order to differentiate the infant with hydrocephalus from the normal infant with a big head (Fig. 24).

Untreated hydrocephalus leads to permanent brain injury, therefore surgical treatment should be prompt. The usual practice is to bypass the obstruction by inserting a Spitz–Holter or a Pudenz valve. This is a catheter with a one-way valve, one end of which is inserted into the lateral ventricle whilst the other is passed via the inter-

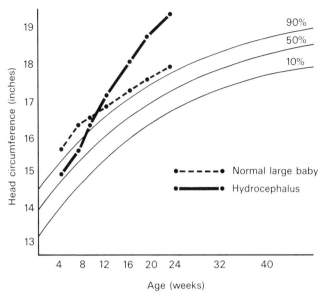

Fig. 24. The head circumference of a normal large baby increases at a rate parallel to the percentile lines; that of the hydrocephalic increases at an abnormal rate.

nal jugular vein into the right atrium (Fig. 25) or into the peritoneal cavity. Depending on the cause of the obstruction and the speed of treatment, normal brain development and function is possible. Low grade infection and other technical problems often prevent the valves from being as permanently effective as desired.

SPINA BIFIDA

This is a common and important congenital defect resulting from failure of closure of the posterior neuropore, which normally occurs around the 27th day of embryonic life. It occurs more commonly amongst whites (Europeans and Americans) than amongst Negroes, and is more frequent in families living in poor socio-economic circumstances.

The commonest and most severe form is a *meningomyelocele* (myelocele) in which elements of the spinal cord

Fig. 25. Pudenz valve draining CSF from the lateral ventricle into the right atrium.

and nerve roots are involved. It may occur at any spinal level but the usual site is the lumbar region. The baby is born with a raw swelling over the spine in which the malformed spinal cord is either exposed or covered by a fragile membrane. The cord is at risk of further damage from infection, drying out or other direct physical trauma (Fig. 26).

The majority are associated with hydrocephalus, particularly as a result of the Arnold–Chiari malformation in which a tongue of malfomed medulla and cerebellum protrudes down through the foramen magnum.

The main physical problems from meningomyelocele are:

1 Legs—partial or complete paralysis below the level of the lesion, with associated sensory loss. Secondary hip

Fig. 26. Meningomyelocele, shortly after birth.

dislocation and leg deformities occur, especially talipes (club foot).

2 Head—associated hydrocephalus with possible brain damage.

3 Bladder—neuropathic bladder with overflow incontinence and recurrent urinary tract infections leading to kidney damage.

In addition, paralysis of the anus will be present if the relevant spinal cord segments or roots are involved. The emotional and social problems for the child and family are massive, varying from the frequent hospital admissions and attendances to the problems of providing suitable education for a paraplegic deformed child.

The policy of earlier years, in which all children with a meningomyelocele had the defect closed by surgery as early as possible, has been replaced by a more selective policy. Surgical treatment is not advised if the baby has gross hydrocephalus, kyphosis, severe paralysis or associated gross congenital anomalies or birth injury. Therefore, it is essential that any baby with the lesion is transferred at once to a centre where expert assessment can be performed and surgical closure attempted when appropriate. This will protect the cord from further damage. Subsequently, the child may be helped by neurosurgical treatment of associated hydrocephalus. Orthopaedic procedures may improve function, especially of the hip. Intermittent or continuous catheter drainage of the bladder may allow continence and prevent kidney damage, but sometimes a urinary tract diversion operation is necessary to create drainage of urine into an ileal conduit. The therapeutic programme is therefore formidable, and the majority are still handicapped at the end.

Meningocele

These are less common and less serious. The sac of CSF is covered by meninges and skin and contains no neural tissue.

Encephalocele

Encephaloceles are protrusions through the skull usually in the occipital region. They are uncommon, and if large are likely to be associated with severe brain damage.

Spina bifida occulta

This is of little importance. Although there is failure of fusion of the posterior neural arches of the vertebrae, the membranes and cord do not project through it and are nearly always normal. The site of the cleft may be marked externally by a naevus, or a tuft of hair. There are usually no neurological disturbances. In 10% of children, X-rays show a gap in the neural arch, but many of these have cartilaginous fusion rather than spina bifida occulta.

Prediction of abnormality

Parents who have had one child with spina bifida have a ten times increased chance of another such child. Biochemical tests have been developed to predict the occurrence. Normal amniotic fluid contains a small amount of alpha-fetoprotein derived from the fetus. If the fetus has anencephaly (an absent skull vault and deformed brain), spina bifida or certain other major abnormalities, the amniotic fluid usually contains a great excess of alpha-fetoprotein. Amniocentesis about the 4th month of pregnancy followed by analysis of the fluid, can be used as a predictive test and possible indication for termination of pregnancy. The reliability of the maternal alpha-fetoprotein blood level as a screening test is being evaluated.

CEREBRAL PALSY

Cerebral palsy is a disorder of posture and movement resulting from a non-progressive lesion of the developing brain. In general the term is rarely applied to brain lesions incurred after the age of 2 years. Children with cerebral palsy are sometimes called 'spastics', but not all have spasticity (see below). It occurs approximately once in every 300 live births.

The main *causes* can be classified according to the time they occur.

1   Intrauterine: genetic, infections such as rubella and toxoplasmosis, and massive irradiation.

2   Perinatal factors are the commonest cause: birth trauma, anoxia, hypoglycaemia, hyperbilirubinaemia.

3   Illness of infancy account for 10% of cerebral palsy: meningitis and encephalitis, trauma and vascular accidents.

Low birth weight is an important associated factor, for one-third of all children with cerebral palsy were low birth weight babies.

The *presentation* varies according to the severity. In the most severe cases poor sucking or altered muscle tone may arouse suspicion soon after birth. More often cerebral palsy is first suspected around the age of 6 months when the child's motor development is delayed—he may have poor head control or be late at sitting. It is important to realise that although the brain lesion is fixed and non-progressive, the disorder it causes varies in the early years as different movement patterns are acquired. Thus an affected infant is often floppy and hypotonic up to the age of 6 months and then becomes hypertonic.

There are three main *types of cerebral palsy*. In the spastic cerebral palsies one or both cerebral hemispheres are damaged. In the dyskinesias (involuntary movements) the basal ganglia are abnormal.

1 Spasticity. Defined as a persistent increase of stretch reflexes resulting in increased tone which is found only in one direction of joint movement ('clasp-knife'). Stretch produces a feeling of increased muscular resistance which characteristically may lessen abruptly ('catch and give reaction'). It is still present during sleep. Tendon reflexes are increased and clonus may be present. The spasticity may be sub-classified according to the limbs involved:

Quadriplegia—of four limbs (Fig. 27). Other terms also are applied to this state: tetraplegia, diplegia (a term introduced by Sigmund Freud to describe spasticity which is more marked in the legs than in the arms) and double hemiplegia (when the arms are worst affected).

Hemiplegia—arm and leg of the same side.

2 Involuntary movements. Choreoathetosis, a mixture of choreic and athetoid movements, is commonest. These irrepressible movements are exacerbated by voluntary movement, and are absent during sleep. They are frequently associated with dystonia (disordered posture with varying hypo- and hypertonicity).

3 Ataxia. This unsteadiness of normal movements is often associated with incoordination, intention tremor and poor balance. Cerebellar lesions are a common cause.

Some children have mixed disorders incorporating features from two or even three of these types of cerebral palsy.

Management

The management of these children is a difficult art. Early comprehensive assessment is essential, firstly because the factors which cause cerebral palsy may cause other

Fig. 27. A 3-year-old boy with spastic quadriplegia. His hips are flexed and adducted, and his arms still show the asymmetric tonic neck reflex.

serious defects, e.g. mental handicap or epilepsy, and secondly because disordered movement can lead to secondary problems, e.g. joint deformities or home and educational problems. Therefore apart from a detailed history and general examination the following have to be assessed: vision, hearing and intelligence, and the emotional and social state of the child and home. The fact that the divorce rate of parents with cerebral palsied children is higher than for any other condition is just one expression of the great stress which such children may place on the family. It is a degree of stress that can be considerably reduced by an energetic and compassionate doctor. Early physiotherapy aims to establish a normal pattern of movement by facilitating normal postural reflexes and inhibiting the awkward persisting primitive reflexes. It also aims to prevent deformity. Orthopaedic surgery can help to prevent and correct deformity in spastic cerebral palsy.

Prognosis

This depends mainly on the presence or absence of associated handicaps, and in particular on the intelligence of the child. With normal intelligence the problems of even the most severe motor handicaps may be overcome. The quality of the management itself affects the prognosis. A severely affected child may require education in a special school where expert physiotherapy, occupational therapy, teaching and other facilities are available.

Children less severely affected manage at normal school, and the least severely affected of all do not always reach the specialist. Their clumsiness, their inability to march in step, or their difficulty in copying shapes may make them an object of derision at school without it being realised that they are suffering from 'minimal brain damage'.

SPACE-OCCUPYING LESIONS

These cause raised intracranial pressure as a result of their own size and by interfering with normal CSF drainage. Headache, misery and irritability are common early symptoms and are followed by unsteadiness, vomiting and visual disturbances. Fits may occur.

In infancy the anterior fontanelle is tense and the skull sutures widened. Tapping the skull may yield a 'cracked pot sound'. In older children papilloedema occurs early. Skull X-ray may show 'copper-beaten' bones with widened sutures and erosion of posterior clinoids. The most important space occupying lesions are:

1 Neoplasm (p. 239).

2 Cerebral abscess

Focal infection in the brain arises from
1   Extension of chronic otitis media.

2 Congenital cyanotic heart disease.
3 Infected emboli from the lungs or elsewhere in the body.

There is a slow invasive stage during which the child is feverish and complains of headache, followed a week or two later by dramatic features of raised intracranial pressure and focal neurological signs. The CSF at first shows a sterile leukocytosis and later a raised protein also. The ESR is always elevated, but there is not always a peripheral blood leukocytosis. The commonest pathogens are streptococci or staphylococci, and early antibiotic treatment can lead to complete cure; but once formed and encapsulated the abscess may only subside after neurosurgical drainage.

3 Subdural haematoma

Bleeding into the subdural space is usually caused by trauma. Subdural haematomata are commonest under the age of 2, in contrast to cerebral abscesses which are uncommon in infancy. Nowadays one of the most important and common causes of subdural haematoma is deliberate violence—the battered baby syndrome (p. 280). The symptoms may present acutely or chronically. The latter are more difficult to diagnose for the traumatic episode may be several weeks past, and the infant may have relatively non-specific features of failure to thrive, low-grade fever and convulsions. Unless it is drained the haematoma may enlarge as the blood breaks down and more fluid is absorbed into the sac. In this way signs of an expanding space-occupying lesion develop and permanent brain damage may occur. Neurosurgery is then urgently required.

CRANIOSYNOSTOSIS (Craniostenosis)

Premature fusion of one or more of the skull sutures results in an unusual-shaped head and may compress the brain or cranial nerves. The prognosis depends upon which sutures are affected. Premature fusion of all sutures results in a bulging forehead, proptosis and brain compression which requires urgent surgery. Premature fusion of a single suture causes a misshapen head which may require surgery for cosmetic reasons. The cause is unknown. Sometimes there is a hereditary factor, and frequently there are associated skeletal abnormalities. The diagnosis is confirmed by skull X-ray.

Skull asymmetry is common in early infancy, but the sutures and fontanelles are normal; one side of the forehead and occiput are displaced forward. The asymmetry becomes less with growth and does not cause problems. There may be associated chest asymmetry. The skull asymmetry is often referred to as *plagiocephaly*, but this term is more properly reserved for asymmetrical craniosynostosis.

ACUTE INFECTIOUS POLYNEURITIS

This is an uncommon condition chiefly affecting children aged 2–10. It is characterized by degeneration of the peripheral nerves and nerve roots. The cause is unknown though it tends to occur shortly after various acute infections. There is an ascending paralysis which in the space of a few days progresses to a symmetrical peripheral neuritis with motor loss, sensory loss and absent tendon reflexes. Provided that the child can be nursed through the acute stage complete recovery gradually occurs.

The CSF is either normal or shows a high protein but normal cell count (Guillain–Barré syndrome).

PROGRESSIVE BRAIN DISEASE

This rare occurrence can be caused by a variety of conditions, many of which are genetically determined. It presents with the loss of previously acquired skills. The end result of progressive neurological degeneration is severe wasting and death, usually from a respiratory infection.

The progressive diseases can be grouped into those which mainly affect the grey matter (e.g. the lipidoses such as Tay–Sachs disease) or the white matter (e.g. metachromatic leucodystrophy). Precise diagnosis may be difficult. It is an important aim because a few conditions may be helped by treatment, and for the majority which cannot be improved, an accurate diagnosis allows genetic counselling for the parents.

Further reading

Gordon N. Paediatric Neurology, *Clinics in Developmental Medicine and Child Neurology*, no 58/59. Heinemann.

O'Donohoe N. *Epilepsies of Childhood*. Butterworth.

Stark G. D. *Spina Bifida*. Blackwell Scientific Publications.

Woods G. E. *The Handicapped Child*. Blackwell Scientific Publications.

Chapter 7

Neuromuscular Disorders

The two main paediatric problems are myopathies—rare in practice but common in examinations, and floppy infants—common in practice but rare in examinations.

MYOPATHIES

Any disorder of skeletal muscle in which the nervous system is normal can be called a myopathy.

The muscular dystrophies

These are an important group of progressive disorders which are usually familial and present in childhood. They are classified according to their distribution, severity of weakness and inheritance:

1   *Duchenne*

The pelvic girdle is severely affected, and proximal muscles more than distal. It presents as a waddling gait or difficulty in climbing stairs. There is often marked lumbar lordosis (Fig. 28). Some children develop enlargement of the calves and other muscles ('pseudohypertrophy'). Knee jerks are absent. This is the commonest type of progressive muscular dystrophy and is also the commonest sex-linked recessive disease in Britain. Affected boys lose the ability to walk about the age of 10 years and tend to die of pneumonia or myocardial involvement in their late teens. A proportion have intellectual impairment. They have a grossly elevated serum creatine phosphokinase level which is present from birth. Most female carriers have a moderately raised level.

Fig. 28. Duchenne dystrophy. There is pseudohypertrophy of the calves, marked lumbar lordosis and winging of the scapula.

2 Limb girdle

This starts in either the shoulder or pelvic girdle. The commonest form of inheritance is autosomal recessive, though the Becker type is sex-linked recessive like Duchenne. Deterioration is slower than with Duchenne dystrophy.

3 Facio-scapulo-humeral

This is the mildest of the three and a normal life span is possible. Autosomal dominant inheritance is usual.

There is no specific cure for progressive muscular dystrophy; therapy is supportive but there should be active physiotherapy to prevent contractures and deformity. Any child with a problem of movement should be encouraged to keep slim. Because of the many variants and the various forms of inheritance a precise clinical diagnosis is important in order to provide reliable genetic counselling for the immediate family and other relatives. Serum enzyme determinations, electromyography and muscle biopsy together with the clinical picture usually provide an accurate diagnosis.

THE FLOPPY INFANT

Infantile hypotonia is a common problem. Extreme examples are noticed because of paucity of movement; but it is commoner for it to present because of poor head control or the feeling on the part of an experienced mother or nurse that the baby is floppy. It is floppy to handle, and when picked up under the arms the baby tends to slip from one's grasp, and its arms are pushed upwards. The feet can be made to touch the ears easily.

Floppy infants can be divided into two main groups:

1 *Paralytic*

In the paralytic there is severe weakness accompanied by hypotonia. These infants make few movements and may be unable to raise their arm upwards against gravity.

It may be caused by a number of rare disorders, including spinal muscular atrophy. There are several distinct types of spinal muscular atrophy, mostly due to autosomal recessive genes. The earlier the onset of symptoms the more rapid the progress and the worse the prognosis. The most severe variety is Werdnig–Hoffmann disease in which progressive degeneration of the anterior horn cells leads to increasing weakness and death in infancy.

2 *Non-paralytic*

There is hypotonia but only mild weakness in the non-paralytic. This is the commoner type of floppy infant.

In these children it is essential to search carefully for the primary condition causing the hypotonia. The possible causes are numerous:

Severe mental retardation.

Cerebral palsy—many children who subsequently show spastic diplegia are floppy in early infancy.

Metabolic disorders—coeliac disease, rickets, scurvy, glycogen storage disease.

Certain syndromes—mongolism, Marfan's syndrome, osteogenesis imperfecta.

Benign congenital hypotonia. The hypotonia is present in the neonate and may be severe. It does not progress and after a period of several months slow improvement leads to complete recovery in most children. A few are found to have congenital myopathy (which has a characteristic biopsy appearance), and these are usually left with mild muscle weakness.

Floppy infants present a difficult diagnostic problem. If no generalised primary cause is apparent a large number of investigations may be needed including serum creatine phosphokinase, electromyography and muscle biopsy.

Further reading

Dubowitz V. *The Floppy Infant.* Spastics International Medical Publications.

Chapter 8

Mental Handicap

There is a continuous spectrum of intelligence from exceptional brilliance to a level too low to be measured by tests. Children with mental handicap (mental subnormality) are conventionally divided into two groups for educational purposes: the severely and moderately educational subnormal, ESN(S) and ESN(M). The intelligence quotient (IQ) is a useful guide to initial educational placement. Children with intelligences on the borderlines between normal and ESN(M), or between ESN(M) and ESN(S) are usually given a trial in the more demanding type of school.

1 *The severely subnormal*

They have an IQ of 50 or less, attend ESN(S) schools and are unlikely to be able to fend for themselves in later life. Associated physical handicaps and congenital abnormalities are common.

2 *The moderately subnormal*

They are the majority (85%) and have an IQ of over 50. They can usually manage in ESN(M) classes and be reasonably independent as adults. Although behaviour problems are common, physical and congenital handicaps are uncommon.

Aetiology

The severely subnormal are scattered throughout all classes and divisions of society, whilst the mildly subnormal are found mainly in families of low intellect and poor social background. It is likely that the poor environment

110

is one of the contributory causes to moderate mental handicap.

Mental handicap may be (1) inborn, or (2) acquired:

1   The inborn or genetic abnormalities result from:
    (a) Chromosome abnormalities, e.g. mongolism.
    (b) Metabolic disease—usually a single gene defect controlled by autosomal recessive inheritance, e.g. phenylketonuria and galactosaemia. These are rare.
    (c) Neurocutaneous syndromes, e.g. tuberose sclerosis (epiloia), and Sturge–Weber syndrome.
    (d) Idiopathic—no cause apparent.
2   Acquired. The brain may be damaged:
    (a) Pre-natally by infection, or more rarely by radiation.
    (b) Perinatally by haemorrhage, anoxia, hyperbilirubinaemia, hypoglycaemia and infection.
    (c) Post-natally by trauma, infection and thyroid deficiency.

Presentation

In the absence of gross congenital abnormalities the mentally handicapped child is likely to present because of slowness at achieving skills. He will usually be slow in all four main fields of development—posture and movement, vision and manipulation, hearing and speech, and social behaviour (p. 72). Sometimes the slowness is marked in everything except posture and movement, because of all the skills a baby acquires, those in the field of posture and movement are least related to intelligence. A careful history is needed. It will usually be found that the child has been slow from early life, perhaps smiling only at 3 or more months of age. The child will have been slow at acquiring new skills and also slow at losing certain responses. Primitive reflexes may have persisted beyond the age of 6 months, or the child may have continued to watch and play with his hands after the age of 6 months (at which age normal children have found more interesting things to do).

The rate of learning should be established. Usually the parents recognize that the child is learning, albeit slowly. Specific questions should be asked to make sure that the child is not deteriorating and losing skills. This is extremely rare but very important as it could be a sign of progressive brain disease (p. 104).

Investigations

The history and physical examination may point to a likely cause. In addition a wide range of special investigations may be needed. These include biochemical investigations of the blood, amino-acid and sugar chromatography of the urine, serological tests for rubella and toxoplasmosis, electroencephalography and neuroradiological studies. One of the reasons for trying to identify the cause is to provide genetic counselling for the parents.

Management

Few causes of mental subnormality are amenable to treatment. Usually the brain damage has to be accepted by the family and the doctor, and every effort concentrated on providing optimal circumstances for the child to develop and learn to the limit of his potential. Many of the causes of mental handicap are known to cause other problems. Some, such as intrauterine rubella, may cause deafness and blindness, others, such as anoxia and hyperbilirubinaemia, may cause cerebral palsy. Therefore any child suspected of having a mental handicap must be comprehensively assessed for associated or secondary handicaps.

Regional child development centres have been established for the comprehensive assessment and treatment of children, together with smaller district centres. These involve many different hospital specialists, as well as education and social service workers of the local authority. The problems of the child and family are identified, and a plan made for aid. The child may need particular specialist aids—spectacles, calipers, or a wheelchair; later on independence training is important. Some subnormal children, particularly those who also have environmental deprivation, will benefit from a developmental stimulation programme. The parents have a continuing need for a sympathetic ear *and* practical help. The concerned doctor checks that they have had, and understand, genetic counselling advice, that they have their full financial allowances, and that they have baby-sitting, child minding or holiday relief accommodation for their handicapped child.

SYNDROMES ASSOCIATED WITH SEVERE MENTAL HANDICAP

Mongolism (Down's syndrome, Trisomy 21)

This occurs approximately once in every 600 births. The mongol child has 47 chromosomes (instead of the usual 46), because of having an extra chromosome 21. It is usually caused by non-disjunction at the time of germ cell formation, and therefore the occurrence of a second mongol child in a family is uncommon. Less than 5% of mongols result from a translocation fault in the parent; such parents may produce other mongol children. The chance of a woman having a mongol child rises steadily after the age of 35. The father's age is irrelevant.

Mongols are recognized by their appearance. They show a variable number of the following features, none of which is pathognomonic, and any of which may be present in a normal child. It is the accumulation of these features which enables a clinical diagnosis to be made (Fig. 29).

The skull is round (brachycephalic) rather than egg-shaped, both face and occiput are flattened. At birth a third fontanelle may be present just anterior to the posterior fontanelle.

The eyes have oblique palpebral fissures, with prominent epicanthic folds. Tiny pale spots (Brushfield's spots) appear on the iris in a ring concentric with the pupil. The eyelashes are scanty, and cataracts, squint and nystagmus common.

The mouth is small and drooping. After infancy the tongue becomes large and furrowed. The pinna may be abnormal.

The neck is short and broad with excess skin posteriorly.

The hands are broad and short. A single transverse palmar crease (simian crease) is common as is a short incurved little finger. The feet have a large gap between

113

Fig. 29. A 5-year-old mongol.

the first and second toes with a longitudinal plantar crease running from that gap.

The mongol shows hypotonicity and hyperextensibility. Developmental progress is delayed in all aspects.

Associated congenital abnormalities are common, particularly congenital heart lesions and duodenal atresia.

Diagnosis

This can usually be made with certainty after examination of the newborn baby. Detailed study of the dermatoglyphics, that is the epidermal ridge patterns of the hands and feet, provides useful confirmatory evidence. Chromosomal analysis is done on the baby if there is uncertainty, and on the parents for genetic counselling.

Progress

Apart from the problem of associated congenital abnormalities, mongol babies may be difficult to feed as infants. Thereafter they tend to be placid and to thrive, though they have an excess of respiratory tract infections. In general they are severely retarded (IQ 25–50) and require education at a school for the severely subnormal. As adults they will require supervision either within the family or in an institution. Their life expectancy is shorter than that of a normal person; they develop the degenerative conditions of old age (arteriosclerosis and malignancy) a decade or two earlier than normal people. Libido is diminished; no mongol is known to have fathered a child, though mongol females have borne children (half of whom are mongols).

Microcephaly

Primary microcephaly is associated with an inadequately developed brain at birth. The head circumference is small and grows abnormally slowly. The fontanelles close early. The infant has a characteristic appearance; the face is normal, but the forehead slopes away so that there is little or no brow to be seen above the face (Fig. 30). Some cases are familial.

Secondary microcephaly is commoner and results from pre- or post-natal damage to the growing brain (e.g. from intrauterine infection or perinatal trauma).

Although the skull circumference and growth may be normal at first, from the time of the brain damage the growth decreases and microcephaly develops. The proportions of the face and skull are relatively normal.

Fig. 30. An 8-month-old infant with primary microcephaly.

N.B. Craniosynostosis (p. 103) is a disorder of bone fusion in children with potentially normal brains and intelligence, and results in heads of bizarre shape.

Further reading

Woods G. E. *The Handicapped Child*. Blackwell Scientific Publications.

Chapter 9

Emotional and Behavioural Problems

The requirements for normal physical and mental growth have been described in Chapters 3 and 4. This chapter is about the child's emotional growth, the things which may disturb it, and the ways in which this disturbance may show itself. At what age in childhood can one begin to talk about the emotions? Some newborn babies cry a lot, others are placid, but there is no way of knowing whether their different behaviour indicates physical or emotional differences. Sudden loud noises or being dropped may elicit a 'startle' response in newborns, but one cannot tell whether they feel frightened. At 1–2 months the infant begins to become socially responsive, and if a smile is assumed to equate with a pleasurable sensation, one can begin to study emotional reactions.

Probably the most important need for healthy emotional development in the early years of life is constancy. The more widely used term, security, really only means that-which-makes-the-child-feel-secure, and leaves one wondering what it is. A close, personal and physical relationship with one person who provides food, warmth and comfort appears to be the earliest essential. Normally this will be mother, but on occasions it may be father, grandmother, foster-mother, or some other mother substitute. Initially the infant is aware only of mother, but as he grows he absorbs siblings, father and others into his world and begins to establish relationships with them. His horizons expand from mother to family to neighbourhood to school and beyond. At each stage there are new situations to explore, new relationships to establish. Each stage is built on the one before, which explains the crucial importance of the earliest stages.

Constancy implies (a) that a person, and later a group, can be relied upon to provide the necessities of life;

(b) that the person or group is constantly available and does not change; (c) that the responses to exploratory activities are constant. It follows that inconstancy arises (a) when the child does not know to whom he should turn; (b) when the composition of the group suddenly changes, or he is suddenly removed from it; and (c) if he receives conflicting responses, for example, in terms of what he may or may not do. If rules are needed for a game of football, how much more so for life. The rules themselves are not so important and will vary from one family to another: but everyone in the family needs to know the rules and to stick to them. In the early months and years the child is putting down his emotional roots. If the ground is for ever being disturbed, the roots cannot grow.

The form which an emotional disturbance takes will depend in part upon the cause and in part upon the child's personality and the family patterns of response to stress. Disorders of eating and sleeping usually result from ill-judged or inconsistent handling by parents. Stress is likely to manifest itself as migraine if the child comes from a headache-prone family. The placid child is unlikely to have temper tantrums but may have recurrent abdominal pain. The toddler who feels challenged by the arrival of a new baby may resort to infantile behaviour.

In summary, the doctor is likely to be faced with two groups of children whose problems are basically emotional. The first comprises those with psychosomatic disorders, in which the emotional stress causes physical symptoms. The second comprises those with overt disorders of behaviour. Psychosis is rare.

STRESS AND ITS SYMPTOMS IN CHILDHOOD

Emotional stresses, in children as in adults, frequently manifest themselves in physical symptoms. These include disease complexes discussed elsewhere: asthma and eczema (p. 207), obesity (p. 56), and ulcerative colitis (p. 184). Emotional disorder can occasionally be life-threatening, as in anorexia nervosa. Far more common are recurrent abdominal pains, headache, vomiting or limb pains as manifestations of stress. Habit spasms (tics), compulsive drinking and sleep disorders in older children are also usually due to psychological stresses.

The kinds of stress that may precipitate symptoms vary enormously, as does the severity of the stress. Some children are of a buoyant temperament and can ride almost any crisis; others are sensitive plants and bow before every emotional breeze. The following is by no means a comprehensive list but includes some of the stresses most commonly afflicting children.

1 Acute separation. The death of a parent or of a much-loved grandparent, emergency admission to hospital or moving house, are examples of acute separations. These are most upsetting to young children around 2–4 years old who are conscious of the separation but unable to understand the reason.

2 Parental discord. All children are conscious of the relationship between their parents and will be aware of any deterioration. When discord develops, the child is likely to be involved and invited to take sides in the contest. This is a devastating experience for all but the most insensitive. A history of recent separation or divorce is not uncommon when children present with stress symptoms, but the symptoms have usually begun long before the break. Indeed, if the marriage is damaged beyond repair a physical separation of the parents may provide the only foundation on which to rebuild the child's security.

3 Inconsistent handling. If a child is permitted something by one parent that is denied by the other; or forbidden by parents but encouraged by grandparents; or punished on one occasion and ignored on another, this is likely to encourage the more flamboyant kinds of behaviour disorder such as temper tantrums, breath-holding attacks, and difficulties with eating and sleeping. The intelligent child is quick to play off one adult against another, or to achieve his own ends by alarming or distressing the adults around him. Diplomacy and blackmail can be learned from an early age.

4 Boredom. If children have time on their hands the effect varies with age. The infant who is deprived of companionship and playthings will be delayed in his

development. Without encouragement and practice, motor skills, speech and social activities lag. The bored toddler who is confined to his cot 'to keep him out of mischief', having thrown all toys overboard, can choose between cot-rocking, head-banging, pulling out his hair (trichotillomania), masturbating or playing with his excreta. Older children who are bored may take to truancy and vandalism.

5   Sibling rivalry. Toddlers are expected to be jealous of their new baby brothers and sisters. In fact, most toddlers, and especially first-borns, delight in the new baby, but may resent the time which his mother devotes to it. If there is regression or aggression, it is likely to be directed against the mother rather than against the baby. When the new baby is old enough to be mobile and to interfere with the elder sibling's activities jealousy will become more obvious. At school age, constant comparisons between siblings with different capabilities and interests can devastate the less clever or the clumsy. It is almost unbelievable how many parents will discuss their children in their presence, as if they were not there, drawing unfavourable comparisons with other children. This may lead to anti-social behaviour such as lying, stealing, truancy or wanton destruction.

6   Great expectations. Closely allied is the unfavourable comparison between the child's achievements at school and the expectations of his parents or teachers. Parents naturally want their child to do well but may form an unrealistic idea of his capabilities or set their hearts on a career for him which he could never achieve. Although many a child 'could do better if he tried', not everyone is destined for an honours degree. If parents constantly nag when he is doing his best, psychological breakdown will follow. Recurrent abdominal pain, if it leads to school avoidance, may be the presenting symptom, or there may be more serious disturbance, e.g. anorexia nervosa.

7   Acute emotional shock. Sometimes a child is witness to, or involved in, an acutely distressing situation—a road accident, a sudden death, or assault of a young girl. Such an incident may lead to hysterical symptoms (e.g. mutism), to disturbed behaviour (e.g. night terrors), or to acute physical symptoms (e.g. asthma).

PERIODIC SYNDROME

Stress may manifest as recurrent abdominal pains, headaches, limb pains, vomiting or other symptoms. Many descriptive terms have been used—abdominal migraine, bilious attacks, acidosis, cyclical vomiting—and the term 'periodic syndrome' is used to include all recurrent symptoms or symptom-complexes attributable to stress. They are common.

Recurrent abdominal pain is by far the most common of these symptoms, and it has usually persisted for a year or more by the time medical advice is sought. The pain is almost always central abdominal, does not radiate widely, and may be associated with nausea. It can be quite severe, the child becoming quiet and pale. It occurs at any time of day, without obvious precipitating cause, but scarcely ever wakes the child at night. The child may complain of pain several times in a week and then not at all for a month or two. As children with recurrent abdominal pain are usually of school age, the parents often suspect some stress at school. The class teacher, whose report is often helpful, suspects some tension at home and is very often right.

Careful clinical examination, including microscopy of the urine, supported if necessary by IVP or barium meal, must be carried out to exclude organic causes of abdominal pain, and to provide a basis of reassurance for the parents. Constipation can cause pain, usually a pelvic discomfort relieved by defaecation. Rarely, abdominal pain may be the sole symptom of temporal lobe epilepsy. This would be suggested by a history of sleep following the pain, an abnormal EEG, and a good response to anticonvulsants. Recurrent abdominal pain is sometimes the presenting symptom of coeliac disease or of food allergy (especially milk).

Headache is a common stress symptom in children. It is usually frontal, sometimes vertical or occipital. It may be unilateral (migraine) and associated with nausea or vomiting, but a visual aura is much less common in children than in adults with migraine. In most cases, headache is the family stress symptom, and one or both parents will admit to migraine or sick headaches. Migraine sometimes results from food sensitivity (chocolate, cheese).

Vomiting is intimately connected with the emotions ('I'm sick of it all') but is less common than pain as a stress symptom. It occurs at a younger age than recurrent pains. As young children readily become ketotic and ketosis can cause vomiting, a vicious circle may develop.

After listening to the history, there are two useful supplementary questions. 'What sort of a boy/girl is he/she?' Children with stress symptoms are far more often described as nervous, worriers, perfectionists or solitary than as placid, happy-go-lucky or gregarious. 'Where does this temperament come from?' usually elicits a rueful smile and the admission that one or both parents are cast in the same die. This helps understanding. Examination reveals no disease, but bitten fingernails may indicate the tension behind the smile.

It is not to be expected that stress symptoms will be spirited away, but much can be given by the exclusion of organic disease (especially the mythical grumbling appendix), by explanation of the nature of the symptoms and by encouragement not to pay *undue* attention to them. It is also wise for the doctor to make clear that he understands that the pains are real and not imaginary. Every effort should be made to identify stresses, and health visitors and teachers can be very helpful here, but often the symptom is being perpetuated by parental anxiety, in which case a careful history and examination coupled with firm reassurance may be all that is needed. Drugs should be avoided.

ENURESIS

Enuresis is a common problem. The term is used to describe inappropriate voiding of urine at an age when control of micturition would be expected. Children learn to be dry by day at about 2 years, and by night at about 3 years. By $3\frac{1}{2}$ years 75% of children are dry by day and night. Most children who wet have 'intermittent' enuresis; it is exceedingly rare to encounter children of school age with true 'primary' enuresis, (i.e. who have never had a dry night). 'Secondary' or onset enuresis refers to the situation when a child who has been dry for at least 1 year starts wetting again. Bed wetting (nocturnal enuresis) is a much commoner problem than daytime wetting (diurnal enuresis).

At 5 years 15% of children wet their beds, by 10 years the figure is down to 5% and at 15 years 1%. *Nocturnal enuresis* is commoner in boys and in lower social classes. Its origins are multiple, and in any child may result from several factors. A genetic predisposition, with a positive family history, is common. Developmental delay may be a factor; just as some children are late walking so some are late at learning to control micturition. Stressful events at the time when the child was learning to get dry may interfere with the learning process and severe stress later in childhood sometimes causes a relapse of enuresis. Most enuretic children do not suffer from either a psychological illness or an organic illness.

Organic causes for bed wetting, such as diabetes mellitus or an ectopic ureter, are very rare. However, the child with enuresis should have a full physical examination, if only to reassure the parents who may be convinced that a disease is the cause. If as is usual the child has had a few nights completely dry one can be sure that there is no defect in the mechanics of the urinary tract such as ectopic ureter or neuropathic bladder. The urine should be tested for glucose, and for infection since urinary tract infection is more common in enuretic children.

Management of the enuretic child is a rewarding art. It is a condition which will go and in most cases an enthusiastic doctor can accelerate the natural cure. Concern and time to listen and explain are vital. Sometimes the home situation with the mother spending the days washing the sheets and the nights changing them is so tense that the general atmosphere of stress and bad temper increases the wetting. Simply explaining to the parents that 1 in 8 of other 5-year-old children also wet the bed will help greatly, and the child will be comforted to learn that at least 3 others in his class wet their beds. Punishment has no place: the children are anxious, indeed over-anxious, to stop wetting. Rewards and encouragement may help. The child can be given a notebook, diary or chart in which to stick coloured stars after a dry night. This chart also helps the doctor assess progress. If the child micturates frequently during the day (has a small functional bladder capacity) the child can be trained to hold on for longer to get the bladder used to a larger urine volume. Drugs may be of temporary help particularly if the doctor believes in them and makes that belief clear to the parents and child. Imipramine appears to be the most successful. Conditioning therapy by enuresis alarm is increasingly used, and has a high success rate. The alarm is fitted to the child's bed and goes off when the child has wet; within 3 months' use most children either awaken before they wet (and go to the lavatory) or sleep through without wetting.

Diurnal enuresis (day-time wetting) is usually associated with nocturnal enuresis, but it may occur independently. The usual problem is dampening of the pants rather than puddles of urine on the floor. It is particularly common in girls and is usually associated with urgency of micturition. It may be caused by, as well as a possible cause of, urinary tract infection. Therefore, if a school-child has day-time wetting it is important to check the urine carefully for infection. Treatment of the infection sometimes lessens the wetting. In schoolboys day-time wetting tends to be associated with soiling and more overt behaviour disturbance.

DISTURBANCE OF BOWEL HABIT

Potty training may be started any time in the first 2 years, and a few parents choose to defer it for longer. If started very young, it is the parents who are training themselves to put a pot under the baby when he is going to pass faeces or urine, most commonly after a feed. This helps to establish a conditioned reflex, reinforced by praise when something arrives in the pot but *not* by punishing the reverse. Toddlers should not be left sitting on their pots for long periods, nor should potty-training be obsessional or coercive ('You can't until . . .', or, 'unless . . .'). Faulty bowel training predisposes towards constipation which may become life-long.

Disturbances of bowel habit in children comprise:
(a) Chronic constipation, which may be complicated by faecal soiling.
(b) Faecal incontinence resulting from neurological disorders (e.g. meningomyelocele).

(c) Encopresis: deliberate defaecation in inappropriate places.

(d) Recurrent diarrhoea of toddlers (p. 167).

Faecal soiling, which is most common at 5–10 years, begins as constipation leading to faecal retention. Sometimes this has been 'deliberate', starting during a negativistic phase of development and precipitated by coercive bowel training. Sometimes a hard stool has caused anal fissure, an acutely painful condition which inhibits defaecation and increases constipation. At other times inadequate parental supervision has resulted in infrequent and incomplete bowel actions. The rectum becomes distended with impacted faeces right down to the anal margin. In extreme cases only liquid matter can escape, causing spurious diarrhoea with faecal soiling, of which the child is unaware. His school companions, by contrast, are only too well aware of it, and the child with soiling may become a social outcast.

The abdomen contains hard, faecal masses, often filling the lower half of the abdomen. Rectal examination reveals faeces right down to the anus. There is unlikely to be confusion with Hirschsprung's diseases which usually presents at a much earlier age and in which obstruction is only exceptionally as low as the anus. Unless there is real diagnostic doubt, a barium enema is best avoided.

Management involves first the thorough emptying of accumulated faeces by enemata: suppositories are rarely adequate, and manual removal under anaesthesia is sometimes needed. Bowel training must then be instituted by regular toileting and the use of faecal softening agents such as disodium sulphosuccinate. Laxatives are often needed initially. The addition of fibre (e.g. bran) to the diet is often helpful. Instant success is not to be expected because the rectum takes time to resume its normal calibre and sensation. Admission to hospital for 3–4 weeks is helpful if home management fails.

Encopresis is a symptom of serious psychological upset and the advice of a child psychiatrist should be sought.

HABIT SPASMS (TICS)

Repetitive, involuntary movements, involving particularly the head and neck, may occur in response to emotional stress. Tics are not rhythmical and cannot be stopped voluntarily. They are most frequent in boys aged 8–11 years. There may have been a reason for the movement initially—a twist of the neck in a tight collar, a toss of the head when the hair fell over the eyes—but the movement persists when the reason has gone. Entreaties (or threats) to the child to desist only serve to make it worse. Frequent blinking is usually a symptom of stress rather than an indication of any ocular disease. The only possible diagnostic confusion is with chorea, which is a rare disease (p. 196).

SLEEP DISORDERS

Sleepless children demoralize parents. Young children are demanding by day, but parents survive if they can enjoy peaceful nights. Sleeplessness may begin for a good reason, but persist as a bad habit. Children differ in their personalities from birth. Some seem to be born 'difficult' while others are placid.

Young infants sleep most of the time and crying usually indicates hunger, thirst, cold or pain. It is difficult to be sure of the emotional needs for sound sleep at this age, but the infants of anxious or depressed mothers often seem to be tense and cry readily. A period of wakefulness during the day is common in early infancy (see 3-months colic, p. 48).

The most difficult sleep problems are usually seen in toddlers. Some do not settle down when put to bed: others sleep for a few hours and are then full of activity when the rest of the household is sound asleep. By the time advice is sought these habits have usually persisted for a long time and parents have tried both protracted and complicated bed-time routines, and the almost irreversible step of admitting the child to the parental bed. It is always noticeable that whilst the parents often look worn out, the offending child has boundless energy.

This problem can often be traced to one of two sources. It may date from an illness or upset in which a few broken nights were to be expected, but has been protracted by over-solicitous attention. Toddlers are not stupid and soon recognize when they are on to a good thing. The other common cause is putting the child to bed too early or at no fixed time. Children vary enormously in their sleep requirements and sometimes seem to need less than their parents. If put to bed early, either because they are thought to need so many hours' sleep or because parents like a little time together in the evening, they are wide awake and resent being confined to a cot.

Sleep problems are best prevented by a sensible routine and a firm line when unreasonable demands are made. Before resorting to drugs it is worth trying simple remedies. If the child is fearful of the dark, a night light or open door to a lit landing may bring calm. If the child demands the presence of mother until asleep, he may accept instead an article of her clothing as a talisman. If bad habits are firmly established temporary use of hypnotics may be unavoidable. Chloral is safe and there are palatable preparations for children. High doses are often needed initially. The right dose (as of any drug) is that which achieves the desired effect.

Nightmares are common at all ages. Parents, having experienced them themselves, are not usually very worried by them. They know that nightmares occur in normal people and that they do not mean major emotional upset. Measures such as leaving the bedroom door open, or a light on, may comfort the child who is frightened of going to bed because of nightmares.

Nightmares occur during rapid eye movement (REM) sleep and are the culmination of a dream adventure, the details of which the child can remember immediately afterwards.

Night terrors are not common, but are most alarming. They occur mainly in the first hour or two of sleep. The child shrieks, sits up and stares wide-eyed and terrified as if being attacked by something only he can see. He may stumble out of bed and seem oblivious to the parents' soothing words. However, within a few minutes he will be sound asleep again and will remember nothing in the morning. The parents can be reassured that night terrors do not indicate serious psychological abnormality, the child does not remember them, and that the child will outgrow them.

Night terrors occur during non-REM sleep, and occur abruptly (not as the result of a dream sequence). They are accompanied by an alarming rise of the pulse and violent respirations which may at times make the parents or doctor suspect an epileptic fit.

Crying Babies

All normal babies cry. Excessive crying, especially at night, exhausts parents and invites physical abuse. Physical causes (e.g. earache) may be responsible for short-term crying. Persistent crying more often reflects household tensions. Mothers who seek advice about excessive crying are often afraid that they or their husbands will lose their tempers and damage the baby. The problem may sound trivial to a busy doctor but *must* always be taken seriously. The health visitor can often help.

BREATH-HOLDING ATTACKS

Known in Yorkshire as 'the kinks,' and by other names elsewhere, breath-holding attacks are common but harmless. They occur in 1–2% of children up to 3 years, and are precipitated by frustration or physical hurt. After one lusty yell the child holds his breath, goes red in the face, and may later become cyanosed and briefly lose consciousness. He then starts breathing again and is soon back to normal. Sometimes cerebral hypoxia is sufficient to cause brief generalized twitching, and the possibility of epilepsy may then be raised. A careful history will usually resolve any doubts. The attacks are benign and self-limiting. The parents require explanation and reassurance. If they can ignore the attacks, this is ideal. If they feel compelled to action, a little cold water over the head (an Anglican baptism rather than total immersion) will relieve the tension all round. Sedatives and tranquillizers are not necessary.

The disorders so far described in this chapter lie within the competence of the general practitioner and paediatrician. Help from psychiatrists, psychologists and psychiatric social workers is usually needed to deal with anti-social behaviour in adolescents and with the more serious behaviour disorders which follow.

SEVERE BEHAVIOUR DISORDERS

Anorexia nervosa

This is uncommon in children, but important. It occurs more commonly in girls than in boys, and rarely before early puberty. In contrast to children who eat poorly because they are depressed, children with anorexia nervosa appear to have an abundance of energy strangely at variance with their microscopic food intake and steadily falling weight. They look ill but insist that they feel well. It is a serious disease which can be fatal, and requires hospital treatment under the supervision of a child psychiatrist.

Autistic behaviour

This incorporates certain characteristics of which the most constant are an avoidance of human contact (especially visual contact), delayed and restricted speech and an obsession with sameness—the same things, the same way, the same ritual. Autistic children prefer things to people and avoid your gaze. Sometimes the onset of symptoms is very early: a mother may say, 'As a baby she would never let me cuddle her.' This sort of behaviour is not uncommon amongst children with mental handicap, deafness, or blindness. *Infantile autism* is autistic behaviour in children without other disability. Such children are often difficult to handle and always difficult to teach because of their inability to communicate. An undue proportion of them come from professional homes, and sometimes one or other parent shows mild autistic features—a preference for solitude, an unwillingness to look you in the eye. The condition is so ill-understood that methods of management (variations on the theme of behaviour modification) are still highly experimental.

Hyperkinetic behaviour

In some ways this is a contrast to autistic behaviour. Children vary greatly in the extent of their spontaneous activities and it is impossible to define the limit between physiological and pathological degrees of over-activity.

Many normal children are 'always on the go', 'never still', and need relatively few hours of sleep. Beyond this is the hyperkinetic syndrome in which these features reach an unreasonable degree. Hyperkinetic children are bursting with restless energy from dawn to dusk, and often much of the night as well. They move their attention from one thing to another in rapid succession and cannot be persuaded to concentrate on anything for more than a few seconds. They are easily distracted and seem incapable of sustained attention. In children of school age this presents a grave educational problem.

The hyperkinetic syndrome is particularly common in children with evidence of brain damage (mental retardation or epilepsy) which further complicates their education. Behaviour modification therapy can help. Amphetamine or methylphenidate may have a paradoxical quietening effect while phenobarbitone often makes things worse.

Further reading

Apley, J., Mac Keith, R. C. and Meadow, S. R. *The Child and his Symptoms*. Blackwell Scientific Publications.

Illingworth, R. S. *The Normal Child: Some Problems of the First Five Years*. Livingstone.

Jolly, H. *The Book of Child Care*. Spier Books.

Chapter 10

The Cardiovascular System

Heart disease in children differs in many important ways from heart disease in adults. Most of it is congenital in origin, most of it is diagnosed before it has caused ill health, and effective treatment can be offered for much of it. Congenital heart disease is not *a* disease, but a multitude of heart defects arising from many causes. Nevertheless it is a useful term covering all heart disease of pre-natal origin. Of every 1000 children born, about 7 have congenital heart disease. The lesions vary in severity from those which are incompatible with life to those which cause no symptoms and require no treatment.

In comparison, all other kinds of heart disease in childhood are uncommon. Rheumatic heart disease varies in frequency with that of rheumatic fever (acute rheumatism). In countries with well-developed social and medical services rheumatic heart disease is rare in children and young adults.

Primary myocardial disease and subacute bacterial endocarditis are rare. Coronary artery disease and essential hypertension, which account for so much adult heart disease, are practically unheard of in childhood.

EXAMINATION OF THE
CARDIOVASCULAR SYSTEM

Although the basic principles of examination of the CVS in children are essentially the same as in adults, there are important differences, especially in infants. The routine examination of the hearts of apparently healthy infants in newborn nurseries and welfare clinics is intended primarily to detect asymptomatic congenital heart disease. The examination of sick infants should include a search for evidence of cardiac failure, which may or may not be due to heart disease.

Cyanosis may be evident at rest or only on exertion, which for the infant means when feeding or crying. In toddlers and older children, minor degrees of arterial desaturation may show as a dark flush on the cheeks, a deceptive appearance suggesting rosy health. Cyanosis due to congenital heart disease is usually associated with clubbing of the fingers and toes, but this is not apparent in the early weeks of life. Breathlessness, like cyanosis, may be evident at rest or only on exertion. It may, of course,

Table 7. Heart Rate and Blood Pressure

	Heart Rate		Blood Pressure			
			Systolic		Diastolic	
Age	Sleeping	Active	50%	95%	50%	95%
Fetus	120–160		—		—	
0–6 months	120	Up to 180	80	110	45	60
3 years	95	120	95	112	64	80
5 years	90	115	97	115	65	80
10 years	80	100	110	130	70	90
15 years	75	100	120	140	70	95

result from non-cardiac disease, but breathlessness on feeding in a small infant is most commonly due to heart disease. The radial pulses are not always easy to feel in babies, but the brachials and femorals should always be palpable. The sleeping pulse rate can often be conveniently counted by observing the pulsations of the anterior fontanelle. The neck veins are not so easy to study in babies as in adults.

Blood pressure measurement is important, but may, at times, be most awkward to measure. Whether by auscultation, palpation or flush method, considerable patience and skill are needed. The child needs to be quiet and at ease. A struggling child will have a high blood pressure. The sphygmomanometer cuff must be chosen with care: too small a cuff yields a false high reading. In a neonate the cuff width should equal half the arm circumference.

For most children the cuff width should be two-thirds the distance between the tip of the shoulder and tip of the elbow. Many of the smaller paediatric cuffs which are necessary for young children are not only narrow but short also. With these cuffs it is imperative to ensure that the rubber bladder lies over the artery which it is to occlude. The cuff width is recorded in the notes alongside the blood pressure. The arm should be at heart level.

Auscultation is the method of choice. This may be difficult in the very young. The Doppler machine for the amplification of blood flow sounds is useful in any paediatric unit, and enables the sounds to be heard with ease in babies. The diastolic pressure should be taken as the muffling of the sound (Korotkoff IV), rather than the disappearance of the tapping sound (Korotkoff V) because in children the sounds often can be heard down to zero.

Palpation of the brachial or radial arteries enables the systolic pressure to be measured when auscultation proves impossible. The flush method is useful in infants and provides a measurement between the systolic and diastolic levels. A cuff of suitable size is applied round the forearm or lower leg and attached to the sphygmomanometer. The hand or foot is then exsanguinated as much as possible either by wrapping Paul's tubing round from distal to proximal or by grasping firmly in the examiner's hand. The cuff is pumped up before compression is released, leaving the extremity blanched. The pressure is then slowly reduced whilst a watch is kept on the pale skin, preferably by a second examiner. The point at which the colour suddenly returns to the skin is the flush pressure.

The position of the apex beat in children can be referred to the nipple line and is normally 1–2 cm outside it, in the 4th or 5th intercostal space. Overactivity of the right ventricle can be detected by palpation in the intercostal spaces just to the left of the sternum and, in infants particularly, in the epigastrium. Hypertrophy of the right ventricle will cause progressive deformity of the chest in young children, with prominence of the lower part of the sternum and the adjacent parts of the costal cartilages. Thrills should be felt for in the suprasternal notch as well as over the praecordium. On auscultation, splitting of the first sound is not uncommon, and of the second sound invariable if the heart and respiratory rates are not too rapid. Splitting of the second sound is wider during inspiration, and often disappears during expiration. Respiration also affects heart rate, causing sinus arrhythmia. This may be so marked in children that the heart rate in inspiration is twice that in expiration, giving the impression of some bizarre disturbance of heart rhythm. Careful observation of respiration and the effect of breath-holding resolve the mystery. The third heart sound is often easy to hear, especially in older children and adolescents. It may be loud enough to masquerade as a diastolic murmur, but comes hard on the heels of the second sound and is of very brief duration.

In addition to the normal heart sounds, innocent murmurs and venous hums are very common in healthy children and are a frequent cause of confusion. The most frequently encountered innocent murmur is an early systolic bruit of squeaky quality (sometimes called 'creaking-gate'), loudest at the lower left sternal edge and often quite loud. It varies with posture (examine standing, sitting and lying) and may disappear on deep inspiration. Another common functional murmur, again systolic, is heard in the pulmonary area and is less easily distinguishable from murmurs of organic origin. A venous hum is a low-pitched, continuous bruit best heard beneath the inner ends of one or both clavicles. It can be altered or abolished by changing the position of the neck.

A precise anatomical diagnosis can rarely be made on clinical grounds alone except by experts. A good quality chest X-ray and an ECG usually provide additional useful information. If there is any question of surgery being considered, further investigation is usually needed to establish the site and severity of obstructions or of abnormal communications. Increasingly, non-invasive investigational techniques such as echo-cardiography are replacing cardiac catheterisation and angiocardiography.

CARDIAC FAILURE

Cardiac failure is a medical emergency. In children it may result from congenital or rheumatic heart disease; from hypertension secondary to renal or other diseases; from acute or chronic respiratory disease; and from other rarer causes. In infancy, severe respiratory infections (pneumonia, bronchiolitis) readily cause heart failure which may be overlooked because the primary disease will cause tachypnoea, tachycardia, crepitations and perhaps cyanosis. The best clue to heart failure in infancy is enlargement of the liver, which may change in size with remarkable rapidity. There will also be tachypnoea and a disproportionate tachycardia (Fig. 31). Pitting oedema is

Fig. 31. Cardiac failure in infancy.

a very late sign of heart failure in babies. It may be anticipated if daily weighing shows a rapid weight gain in a sick infant. Chest X-ray shows an enlarged heart. The management of cardiac failure includes treatment of the cause (where possible) and the administration of oxygen, digoxin and diuretics. Infants are often restless and require sedation; tube feeding may be needed to avoid the effort of sucking; and skilled nursing is essential. The baby is better nursed semi-recumbent. Dosage of digoxin is crucial as the margin between therapeutic and toxic levels is small, and there is no effective antidote. Initial doses of digoxin and diuretics are often best given parenterally. Infants with congenital heart disease awaiting investigation or surgery often need to be maintained on a daily dose of digoxin for months or years.

CONGENITAL HEART DISEASE

Circulatory changes at birth

The ductus arteriosus is, of course, a large, functional vessel in all fetuses. Immediately after birth it closes and the lumen is obliterated over the next few days. The other changes in the circulation at birth include the closure of the ductus venosus, and the functional closure of the foramen ovale as a result of the left atrial pressure rising above that of the right (Fig. 32). The precise mechanics of these important circulatory changes have still not been elucidated. The ductus arteriosus is quite often widely patent in babies who have died from any cause within the first days of life.

Aetiology of congenital heart disease

In very few instances of congenital heart disease is the cause known. Among the known causes are:

1 Autosomal trisomy syndromes. Heart lesions are present in about 25% of mongols, and in a high proportion of infants with other autosomal trisomies.

2 Turner's syndrome, in which a minority of patients have coarctation of the aorta or heart lesions.

3 Other genetic syndromes (e.g. Marfan's, Klippel–Feil).

4 Congenital rubella. Infection in the second month of pregnancy is likely to affect the heart, and will often affect the eye, ear and brain at the same time. Rubella may cause many different heart lesions, but patent ductus arteriosus is particularly common. The introduction of rubella vaccine should gradually eliminate this cause of heart disease.

5 Drugs, including anticonvulsants, alcohol and (in the past) thalidomide.

In the absence of any hereditary syndrome, the parents

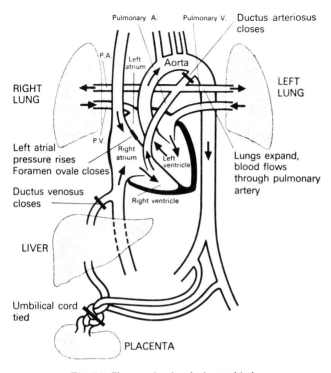

Fig. 32. Changes in circulation at birth.

of a child with congenital heart disease can normally be reassured about the prospects for any further children they may have.

Congenital heart disease, which may involve the heart, the great vessels, or both, can be understood in terms of disordered embryology. Most lesions arise as a consequence of normal embryological processes becoming either arrested before completion, or deviated from their normal course. The consequence is usually either abnormal communication between the systemic and pulmonary circulations, or obstruction to normal blood flow, or a combination of the two. For example, failure of completion of the interventricular or interatrial septa will result in ventricular or atrial septal defects. Failure of division of the truncus arteriosus in the normal way may result in

Fallot's tetralogy, in transposition of the great vessels or in persistent truncus. There may be narrowing of the ventricular outflow tracts, leading to pulmonary or aortic stenosis. The mitral and tricuspid valves are less often involved in congenital lesions, although these two valve rings may remain continuous with one another (persistent atrio-ventricular canal), a lesion which is relatively common in mongols.

Symptoms and signs

The most common symptoms are cyanosis and breathlessness (either at rest or on exertion), difficulty with feeding (which is a form of exertional dyspnoea) and failure to

Table 8. Common congenital heart lesions (these account for 90% of all lesions)

No shunt	Left-to-right shunt	Right-to-left shunt
Pulmonary stenosis	Ventricular septal defect	Tetralogy of Fallot
Aortic stenosis	Atrial septal defect	Transposition of the
Coarctation of the aorta	Patent ductus arteriosus	great vessels

thrive. The most common signs are heart murmurs and evidence of cardiac failure. In general, cyanosis will be present if there is a substantial shunt of blood from the right side of the circulation to the left, but not if there is no shunt or if the shunt is from the left side to the right. Table 8 classifies the principal congenital heart lesions on the basis of the presence and direction of shunt. As the pressure in the left heart and aorta is normally higher than in the right heart and pulmonary artery, an uncomplicated communication between the two sides results in a left-to-right shunt. However, if such a shunt is substantial and is allowed to persist, changes take place in the small pulmonary vessels which lead to pulmonary hypertension and ultimately to a reversal of the shunt. Cyanosis may therefore develop after some years, but should in most cases be prevented by surgical correction of the lesion before the pulmonary vasculature is irreparably damaged.

Left-to-right shunts

Ventricular septal defect

VSD is the commonest congenital lesion. It may affect the upper, membranous part of the septum, the lower, muscular part, or the septum may be virtually absent. The conducting system is hardly ever affected by these lesions. A high VSD may be associated with other lesions (as in Fallot's tetralogy). An isolated defect in the muscular part of the septum (maladie de Roger) is of special interest because it may undergo spontaneous closure. This occurs in at least 20% of cases (possibly in the majority of *small* VSDs) usually within 6–9 months of birth but sometimes appreciably later. In most instances a VSD is recognized by the detection of a heart murmur at a routine examination, either shortly after birth or later in infancy. The murmur is pan-systolic, blowing, sometimes very loud, usually maximal down the left sternal border and often accompanied by a thrill. In symptomless infants there are usually no other abnormal signs. A few infants become breathless on feeding from birth or may go into frank cardiac failure. If tided over their early weeks, they may become symptom-free. Chest X-ray may show a little cardiac enlargement, and increased pulmonary blood flow.

If spontaneous closure does not occur, operative closure may be needed if the shunt is large and pulmonary pressure high. This is an open heart operation and is difficult to undertake in very young children. Pending surgery, digitalization may be required.

Atrial septal defect

ASD may result from failure of closure of the ostium primum or of the ostium secundum. In either case the flow of blood is from the left atrium to the right, so there is no cyanosis. There is a mid-systolic murmur, usually maximal in the second or third interspace to the left of the sternum, and often not as loud or as long as the murmur of a VSD. The second heart sound shows wide splitting which does not vary with respiration. The chest X-ray shows prominence of the pulmonary arc and increased pulmonary vascularity. The ECG often shows incomplete right bundle branch block.

Atrial septal defects seldom close spontaneously and are rarely affected by subacute bacterial endocarditis, but pulmonary hypertension may develop with consequent reversal of the shunt. Ostium secundum defects are high up in the septum and operative closure is relatively simple if the shunt is big enough to warrant it. Ostium primum defects, in contrast, are close to the mitral and tricuspid valves. The valves may themselves be malformed, and attempts to close the defect often lead to distortion and malfunction. There is therefore a very different prognosis for the two main types of ASD.

Patent ductus arteriosus

PDA is the third common lesion characterized by a left-to-right shunt, in this case from the aorta to the pulmonary artery. This is the opposite to the normal blood flow through the fetal ductus. As with septal defects, the lesion is usually diagnosed as a result of a heart murmur being heard at a routine examination in infancy. The murmur is loudest in the pulmonary area, initially systolic but later extending through the second heart sound to become a continuous 'machinery' murmur. This is one of the few murmurs that is absolutely characteristic even to the unskilled ear, and the only common source of confusion is a venous hum. There is usually an accompanying thrill, although this may not be detectable in early infancy, and a high pulse pressure causing a collapsing pulse and visible arteriolar pulsation. The chest X-ray shows a prominent pulmonary arc and increased pulmonary vascularity; these appearances are similar to those seen with ASD, but the physical signs are quite different.

Patent ductus may cause heart failure, pulmonary hypertension, failure to thrive or recurrent chest infections, and may be involved in subacute bacterial endarteritis. Ligation and division is therefore advised and can be carried out whenever necessary. If there is no clinical urgency, it is technically easier when the child is a few years old. In very sick newborns with PDA indomethacin may induce closure, but this treatment is experimental and not without risk.

Right-to-left shunts

The two common congenital heart lesions causing right-to-left shunts and cyanosis ('blue babies') are Fallot's tetralogy and transposition of the great vessels. Both result from abnormal division of the truncus arteriosus. In *transposition*, the septum dividing the truncus has failed to rotate, so that the aorta arises from the right ventricle and the pulmonary artery from the left. This leads to two independent circulations and would be incompatible with survival after birth. In practice, therefore, there is always at least one communication between the two circulations in the form of ASD, VSD or PDA, often two, and sometimes all three. These allow some mixture of oxygenated with deoxygenated blood, sufficient to maintain life, albeit somewhat precariously. Cyanosis and breathlessness, especially on feeding, are conspicuous from birth. A systolic murmur develops but may not be audible for a few days. Chest X-ray shows an enlarged heart, often egg-shaped with the apex of the heart forming the apex of the egg and with a narrow pedicle (because the great vessels lie more directly one behind the other than normal). Pulmonary vascularity is increased.

The mortality amongst infants with transposition used to be virtually 100%, and it is still high. Operative correction is now possible in many cases. The prognosis has also been improved by the ingenious and dramatic manoeuvre of balloon septostomy. If communication between the systemic and pulmonary circulations is very poor, the infant will not survive long enough for surgery even to be considered. It can be improved by the creation of an artificial ASD. A balloon catheter (deflated) is directed through the foramen ovale from the right atrium to the left, the balloon is inflated, and a smart tug on the catheter tears a hole in the atrial septum. The consequent improved oxygenation may ensure the infant's survival for later surgery.

Fallot's tetralogy

Fallot's tetralogy is a single error of development with four consequences. The septum dividing the truncus, instead of joining up with the interventricular septum, deviates to the right. The right ventricular outflow is therefore restricted (pulmonary stenosis or atresia), the aorta extends to the right of the septum (over-riding aorta) and receives blood from both ventricles, and there is a deficiency in the upper part of the membranous septum (VSD). The right ventricle must pump blood either through a narrowed pulmonary orifice or into the aorta in competition with the left ventricle. It does both, but only by increasing its pumping strength (right ventricular hypertrophy). Cyanosis may not be evident at birth but usually becomes noticeable within a few days or weeks, depending upon the degree of right ventricular outflow obstruction. A systolic murmur develops early, and the pulmonary component of the second sound may be weak or absent. Chest X-ray shows right ventricular hypertrophy and diminished pulmonary vascularity.

Unlike transposition, Fallot's tetralogy is compatible with many years of life, though with restricted exercise tolerance. Older children with this lesion may learn the trick of squatting on their haunches to relieve exertional dyspnoea. Operative correction is normally undertaken in two stages, the first to increase the pulmonary blood flow, by creating an artificial ductus arteriosus, and the second, usually before school age, to correct the defects.

Obstructive lesions without shunts

Pulmonary stenosis

This may occur at the level of the valve or of the infundibulum. There is a systolic murmur and thrill in the pulmonary area, and there may be right ventricular hypertrophy. The chest X-ray often shows prominence of the pulmonary arc due to post-stenotic dilatation of the pulmonary artery. If the pressure gradient across the obstruction (as measured at cardiac catheterization) is only slight, no treatment is needed. If it is more severe, valvotomy or infundibular resection will be required.

142

Aortic stenosis

More dangerous is aortic stenosis, because it may limit coronary blood flow whilst increasing the demand by left ventricular hypertrophy, and may therefore lead to early, sudden death. Surgery is less successful than in pulmonary stenosis.

Coarctation

Coarctation varies, anatomically, from a sharply localized narrowing, usually at the point of attachment of the ductus arteriosus, to virtual absence of a length of aortic arch (hypoplastic left heart syndrome). The femoral pulses are weak and delayed relative to the radials, or may be absent unless a patent ductus is feeding the aorta distal to the coarctation, in which case there will be cyanosis of the lower part of the body. The blood pressure is raised in the arms. There is a systolic murmur well heard over the back. It is usually several years before collateral vessels can be detected clinically or radiologically. Results of surgery are good in the short term, less good in the long.

There are very many other congenital heart lesions, and anomalies of the aorta and of the pulmonary veins, of great interest and clinical importance, which may present diagnostic problems. In some of the most severe, murmurs are absent. Specialist help should always be sought sooner rather than later.

General management of children with heart disease

There are two general points relevant to the support given by the doctor to the child with heart disease and his parents: first, the natural anxiety generated by the knowledge (or fear) that the child has a weak heart, and second, the question of restrictions on physical activities. Heart disease equates in the public mind with coronaries, blood pressure, strokes and sudden catastrophes. It probably comes second only to mental and nervous disease in its capacity to induce anxiety. The nature of the child's disability should be explained to the parents in terms which they can understand, and with as much optimism as is compatible with truth. They should be assured that the child will not have heart attacks (except in the rare conditions where this is a possibility) and is not in danger of sudden death. If the child's activities do not need to be restricted, this must be emphasised. The likely time for further investigations and the therapeutic possibilities should be outlined. Ignorance breeds anxiety. It will not do to say 'he has a little heart murmur' and leave it at that. An early specialist opinion will always be appreciated.

Physical activities should not be restricted without good reason. Small VSD's and mild pulmonary stenosis, for example, will not limit cardiac reserve significantly. There is an important difference between competitive activities, in which the determined child may overstretch himself, and non-competitive sports in which he can stop when he tires. The only serious risks are in children with impaired coronary blood flow. Children with congenital heart disease should be given amoxycillin cover for dental extractions to minimize the risk of subacute bacterial endocarditis.

Cardiac arrhythmias

Reference has already been made to sinus arrhythmia which is normal. Paroxysmal tachycardia can occur at any age and in children is often associated with the Wolff–Parkinson–White syndrome. Episodes of bradycardia or cardiac arrest (sick sinus syndrome) may cause loss of consciousness especially on exertion, and may be diagnosed by 24-hour ECG monitoring.

Hypertension

Hypertension is less common in children than in adults; that fact together with the difficulty of its measurement (p. 132) causes it to remain undetected all too often. Blood pressure increases up to the age of 15 when adult levels are reached (Table 7). The mean blood pressure for a 6-month-old of 80/45 rises to 97/65 at 5 years and 110/70 at 10 years. From Table 7 it is clear that a blood pressure of 130/90 in a 5-year-old would be grossly abnormal and, if of sudden onset, it could cause major complications for the child (e.g. heart failure or hypertensive encephalopathy.)

In general those children who have a blood pressure about the 90th centile in early life tend to remain at that end of the distribution curve in later childhood and probably adult life also. The blood pressure of any child has a close correlation with that of the parents and siblings. In childhood, there is no sex difference in blood pressure levels.

The important causes of childhood hypertension are of renal, adrenal (e.g. adrenogenital syndrome and Cushing's syndrome) or vascular (coarctation of the aorta) origin. Renal artery stenosis is exceedingly rare, but renal parenchymal diseases resulting from glomerulonephritis, pyelonephritis, or congenital defect, are relatively common, and are the chief contributors to severe hypertension, hypertensive encephalopathy and retinopathy.

Compared with adults who have hypertension, a primary cause is found much more often, and is itself more often totally correctable. For instance, unilateral kidney disease or coarctation if treated surgically early in life may abolish hypertension. However, 10–15% of children with hypertension do not yield a primary cause, and are then considered to have 'essential hypertension'.

Hypertension may be asymptomatic, or may present in a wide variety of ways—failure to thrive, fits, heart failure or, in the older child, headaches and malaise. Salt restriction, diuretics and hypotensive drugs are used as for adults—and tolerated rather better by most children.

Further reading

Jordan S.C. & Scott O. *Heart Disease in Paediatrics*. Butterworth.

Keith J.D., Rowe R.D. & Vlad P. *Heart Disease in Infancy and Childhood*, Macmillan.

Chapter 11

The Respiratory Tract

The mortality from disorders of the respiratory tract has decreased dramatically in the last 30 years. However, respiratory infections and allergy remain important causes of morbidity and are common reasons for a child being taken to a doctor or admitted to hospital.

Certain problems are more common at certain ages as shown in Fig. 34 (p. 157). The same organism may cause different illnesses at different ages. For example, respiratory syncytial virus, which commonly causes lower respiratory tract illness (bronchiolitis) in infants, is more likely to cause a cold or a sore throat in older children.

Symptoms of respiratory tract disease

Cough in children usually has its origin in the upper respiratory tract (infection, allergy), less often in the lungs. It is usually easy to distinguish a 'throaty' from a 'chesty' cough: a barking cough suggests laryngeal or tracheal disease. Young asthmatics may cough instead of wheeze, especially at night. Children usually swallow their sputum unless it is copious. (Wheezing is discussed on p. 159, stridor on p. 153.)

Earache is common with any upper respiratory catarrh as well as in otitis media. Pain from lower back teeth may be referred to the ear.

Epistaxis (nose bleed) usually originates from the anterior inferior corner of the nasal septum (Little's area). The commonest causes are minor injury and upper respiratory tract infections. The child may alarm everyone by vomiting blood which has been swallowed. Epistaxis may be a prodromal symptom of measles or rubella. First aid consists of sitting the child up and squeezing the nose firmly whilst the child is comforted and told to breathe through the mouth.

UPPER RESPIRATORY TRACT

Examination of the upper respiratory tract

This is an important part of the general examination of any child, especially an ill child. It is difficult in babies, and young children may dislike having their ears examined. Practice makes perfect. The infant is held by the mother as shown in Fig. 33, her hands ensuring that the child's head is secure, so that the speculum cannot accidentally damage the meatus. The pinna is drawn gently upwards and backwards to allow a clear view of

Fig. 33. Mother holding child ready for examination of ears. One hand presses the child's head securely to her chest, the other hand controls the child's outer arm, and presses inwards so trapping the inner arm also.

the ear drum. If wax obscures the view it must be gently removed with a wax hook or cotton wool on an orange stick. If the wax is very hard, softening ear drops may be needed first.

The nose should also be examined with the auriscope, noting the colour of the mucosa, the presence of oedema and secretions.

The mouth must be examined thoroughly and the state of the gums, teeth, tongue and buccal mucosa noted as well as the back of the throat. Older children will on request say 'Ah' and reveal the posterior pharynx. For younger children a good view is sometimes obtained by asking the child to put out his tongue. A wood tongue depressor is well tolerated by most children provided it is used gently and is not placed so far back as to cause gagging. It is difficult to get a good view of the throat in babies. Never use force to view the throat of a young child with stridor: it may precipitate fatal respiratory obstruction.

Upper respiratory tract infections

Most illnesses of childhood are infections; most childhood infections are respiratory; and most respiratory infections involve only the upper respiratory tract. A wide variety of micro-organisms are involved, but the great majority are viral. The terms tonsillitis and otitis media are used if there is clear evidence of inflammation of the tonsils or middle ears respectively. In the absence of tonsils (atrophied or removed) an inflamed throat is called pharyngitis.

The term 'upper respiratory tract infection' (URTI) is conventionally used to describe the equivalent of the common cold in young children. It presents with cough, anorexia and fever. In addition to nasal obstruction, the throat may be congested. Eustachian tube obstruction often causes earache and the eardrums may appear congested. Antibiotics are not indicated, but decongestant nose drops (e.g. $1/4\%$ ephedrine in saline) before feeds will make it easier for babies to suck; aspirin or paracetamol will reduce fever; both will relieve earache.

Infections of the upper respiratory tract are the usual precipitants of febrile convulsions (p. 86) and are sometimes the precursors of acute specific fevers, especially measles (p. 267).

Otitis media

Acute otitis media is common throughout the first 8 years of childhood, and is generally associated with an infection of the nasopharynx. In the older child the cardinal symptoms of earache, discharge or deafness make detection easy. In infants it may not be so obvious. They usually have a high fever and are irritable, rolling their heads from side to side, or rubbing their ears.

At onset there may be just mild inflammation of the pars flaccida (the superior part of the tympanic membrane) with dilated vessels running down the handle of the malleus, and an absent light reflex. This progresses to a red bulging tympanic membrane which may perforate and discharge pus. This should be differentiated from the mildly pink dull drum that may be present in any child with an URTI.

In at least half the affected children the cause will be viral. In the rest the pathogens more frequently incriminated are *Streptococcus pneumoniae* and *Haemophilus influenzae*. Ampicillin is the antibiotic of choice, and aspirin is invaluable for the fever and pain.

Mastoiditis, lateral sinus thrombosis, meningitis, and cerebral abscess are rare complications. Persistent infection or discharge—chronic otitis media—is more common.

Secretory otitis media (glue ear, serous otitis media)

The accumulation of sticky serous material in the middle ear may arise insidiously or following acute otitis media. The symptoms are earache, deafness or a feeling of fullness or 'popping' in the ear. It is especially common in children who have atopy, frequent upper respiratory infections or cleft palate. The eardrum is usually dull and retracted. The malleus handle is more horizontal than usual and appears shorter, broader and whiter. The light reflex may be absent. The mobility of the eardrum as tested by pneumatic speculum is impaired and there is usually conductive hearing loss. The peak incidence is from 5 to 9 years when it is the commonest reason for hearing loss. Antibiotics, antihistamines and decongestant nose drops may be given, but in cases where the fluid is very thick, or there is recurrence, an indwelling tube (grommet) is inserted through the eardrum to aerate the middle ear.

Any child who has otitis media must be followed up until the eardrum and hearing are normal. If response to treatment is slow or infections recur, an ear, nose and throat specialist should be consulted.

Deafness

Hearing exists before birth and can be demonstrated in neonates. They startle to a loud noise, or become quiet in response to a diminuendo growl. An infant's hearing is most easily tested at 8 months of age when the child has an insatiable curiosity for new sounds. All children should be tested at this age using the tests described on page 74. Appropriate tests are available for toddlers. Pure tone audiometry is not usually possible before 3–4 years.

Deafness may originate from pre-, peri- or post-natal factors:

1 Prenatal factors include hereditary deafness, maternal infection (e.g. rubella) and malformations of the ear. Congenital rubella deafness is progressive and may not be detectable for months or years.

2 Perinatal factors include cerebral hypoxia and kernicterus.

3 Postnatal factors include meningitis, encephalitis, otitis media, and ototoxic drugs.

Congenitally deaf babies babble normally for about 6 months but then become quieter, do not talk but communicate by gesture. They may also have temper tantrums or other behavioural problems.

Most deaf children have some residual hearing, and so will be helped by a hearing aid which can be fitted as early as 3 months of age. That is the start of the treatment, not the end. The child requires prolonged exposure to speech and sounds at a level which he can hear with the hearing aid.

Skilled help is needed from a team of otologist, audiologist, hearing-aid technician and specially trained teachers. Education for the deaf can be started from 2 years, but most deaf children will enter the partially hearing unit of a nursery school at 3–4 years and then progress to similar units attached to normal schools or to special schools for the deaf. A few children behave as if deaf but respond to hearing tests normally. Theirs is a problem of auditory discrimination, an inability to interpret sounds.

Tonsils and adenoids

Lymphoid tissue grows rapidly in the first 5 years of life. Tonsils and adenoids are usually small in infants and reach their greatest relative size between 4 and 7 years. Cervical glands are normally palpable at this age, and readily enlarge in response to local infection.

Acute tonsillitis

This is very common in the age group 2–8. It is uncommon in infants. There is sudden onset of fever, sore throat, dysphagia. Vomiting and abdominal pains are common in toddlers. The tonsils are enlarged and fiery red; exudate may appear later. The commonest pathogen to be cultured is beta-haemolytic streptococcus, but no bacterial pathogen can be identified in over half the cases. The presence of small petechiae on the palate or ulcers on the buccal mucosa or gums makes a viral aetiology more likely. Aspirin and plenty of cool drinks provide symptomatic relief. Penicillin is often used because it will eradicate streptococci and reduce the risk of complications.

Complications are rare, but important; they may be immediate or delayed.
1   Immediate complications are:
(a) *Peritonsillar abscess* (quinsy) which is characterised by severe symptoms of tonsillitis and marked dysphagia. The tonsil appears displaced towards the midline with the anterior pillar of the fauces pushed forward.
(b) *Cervical abscess*. Marked cervical adenitis is usual at the time of tonsillitis, but occasionally infection

localises in one of the cervical lymph glands to form an abscess. Early antibiotic treatment of peritonsillar or cervical abscess may produce cure, but once they are fully developed surgical drainage is required.

2 Delayed complications after certain streptococcal infections of the tonsil are:
   (a) *Rheumatic fever* (p. 195) 1–2 weeks after the infection.
   (b) *Acute nephritis* (p. 219) 2–3 weeks after the infection.

Tonsillectomy

This operation is becoming less fashionable. It is reserved chiefly for children over the age of 4 who have had recurrent bouts of acute tonsillitis (more than three a year), or persistent or chronic infection of the tonsils.

Parents seek the operation for a multiplicity of reasons. They need to be told that in general tonsillectomy does not prevent the child catching colds, or getting sore throats or bronchitis; it does not improve the child's appetite or growth. Large healthy tonsils rarely cause any trouble—'Large tonsils need to be removed from the text book and not from the child's throat.'

Adenoidectomy

This is usually done at the same time as tonsillectomy. Indications for it to be done independently are recurrent otitis media, sinusitis or obstruction of the nasopharynx.

Sinusitis

The frontal and sphenoidal sinuses do not develop until 5 and 9 years respectively. The maxillary and ethmoidal sinuses are small in these years and sinusitis is uncommon before the age of 5. Maxillarly antra generally reflect nasal pathology (infection or allergy). Post-nasal drip may cause nocturnal or early morning cough.

Allergic rhinitis

The symptoms are recurrent bouts of sneezing with a

watery nasal discharge and watering eyes which are worse when the child is outside in bright sunshine. The nose may be blocked, and inspection inside the nostril reveals pale oedematous mucosa. When it occurs in late spring and early summer in response to grass pollen, it is called *hay fever*, but it may occur in response to a variety of allergens including dust, animal dander and moulds. A careful history is more likely to identify the allergen than skin testing. Avoidance of the allergen may not be possible. Sodium cromoglycate nose and eye drops are useful; a few children are helped by antihistamines. Desensitising injections given in the winter lessen the incidence and severity of hay fever the following spring.

Stridor

Stridor is noisy breathing originating from above the bronchi. It commonly originates from the larynx and is mainly inspiratory in timing.

The young child's larynx is not only relatively smaller, but the walls are flabby compared with the firm cartilaginous adult larynx. It is a voice bag not a voice box and it collapses and obstructs easily.

Congenital stridor

Stridor caused by abnormalities of the pharynx, larynx or trachea may be audible from birth. The least rare form, 'congenital laryngeal stridor', is due to floppy aryepiglottic folds. It does not cause serious obstruction and gradually disappears as the child grows and the laryngeal cartilage becomes firmer.

Acute laryngotracheitis

This is common from 1 to 4 years, and alarming. There is sudden onset of stridor, harsh cry and a barking cough (croup) which sounds like a performing seal. There is moderate fever and systemic illness. The fauces may be mildly inflamed. In addition to stridor there may be indrawing of the ribs and suprasternal notch if obstruction is marked. A raised respiratory rate and abnormal signs in the lungs suggest that the lower respiratory tract is also involved.

Laryngotracheitis is of viral origin, so antibiotics are not necessary. Cold humidity gives symptomatic relief. Sedation lessens anxiety and may help the breathing.

In *acute epiglottitis,* the swollen epiglottis may be seen like a cherry when the pharynx is examined or may be revealed by a soft-tissue lateral X-ray of the neck. *Haemophilus influenzae* is usually responsible and ampicillin is indicated.

Management of stridor poses a lot of problems because of the danger of serious respiratory obstruction, especially in babies and toddlers. It is not usually difficult to exclude rare causes of acute respiratory obstruction such as diphtheria, or an abscess, gland or tumour compressing the larynx. Laryngeal foreign body is more difficult to exclude, particularly if it is not radio-opaque, though there may be a history of choking. A case can be made for admitting to hospital any child with stridor of sudden onset lest total obstruction develops necessitating tracheostomy. In practice admission is usually confined to those whose stridor is associated with one of the following:

(a) acute epiglottis;
(b) marked respiratory distress;
(c) age under 4 years;
(d) very worried parents.

The stridor usually lessens within 12 hours and has gone within 3 days. If it persists or recurs laryngoscopy is indicated.

Influenza

Influenza tends to occur in epidemics, affecting particularly schoolchildren and young adults. The general symptoms of high fever and malaise tend to overshadow the dry cough and sore throat, though there may be signs of pharyngitis, tracheitis or bronchitis. The main complications result from secondary bacterial infection of the lungs, middle ear or sinuses.

The brief incubation period and high infectivity favour

massive outbreaks in institutions such as boarding schools. The large number of strains, as well as the frequency of mutation involving the three types of myxovirus influenzae, make immunisation of limited value. Treatment is symptomatic.

LOWER RESPIRATORY TRACT

The bronchi and other airways together with the blood vessels supplying them are present by the 20th week of gestation. Thereafter they enlarge but do not reduplicate. In contrast, the alveoli and their blood vessels are relatively few in number at birth. During the next 8 years active production of alveoli raises their number from 20 million to the adult complement of 300 million. Respiratory disease in early childhood may therefore interfere with normal lung development as well as causing direct lung damage.

The airways of an infant are particularly liable to obstruction. A tiny amount of mucus or a small degree of bronchospasm may narrow the airway dangerously, leading to poor oxygenation or collapse or a lung segment.

Examination of the chest

The thoracic cage is more mobile in young children than in adults. In response to airways obstruction the sternum and lower ribs may be sucked in with each inspiration. Chronic airways obstruction with hyperinflation of the lungs causes a prominent sternum and an increased anteroposterior diameter. Frequent episodes of obstruction lead to indrawing of the rib cage along the line of attachment of the diaphragm (Harrison's sulcus).

The respiratory rate rises much more readily than in adults and reflects the severity of the disorder. It must be timed accurately: in infants, who often have irregular breathing, it should be timed over a full minute before the baby is disturbed or undressed. (It is meaningless to time a crying infant's respiration.) The respiratory rate in the neonatal period is 30–40/minute. By the age of 2 months the rate is under 30/minute. A respiratory rate of over 40/minute is abnormal and by far the most likely cause is a respiratory infection. However, one needs to remember the other possible causes for a rapid respiratory rate: heart failure, metabolic acidosis, neurological disease and hysterical overbreathing (in adolescents). Tactile vocal fremitus is of little use in children. Percussion and auscultation are very helpful, but sounds are very freely transmitted in a young child's chest, making localisation difficult. It is important to ensure that coarse crepitations are not in fact noises transmitted from the throat. Bronchial breathing can often be heard over the upper half of a normal child's chest because of direct transmission from the main bronchi.

Lower respiratory tract infections

Bronchitis and bronchiolitis

Acute bronchitis occurs at all ages and is characterised by cough, fever and often wheezing. It is a common early feature of measles and whooping cough. Chronic bronchitis does not occur in children.

Bronchiolitis is confined to infants; the peak age is 4 months. Most cases are caused by respiratory syncytial virus and occur in winter epidemics. Older members of the household merely have mild upper respiratory tract symptoms. Bronchiolitis develops suddenly. In the morning the infant may just be a bit snuffly, but by afternoon he is irritable, coughing and breathless. The respiratory rate is high and, as respiratory distress increases, cyanosis may appear. Widespread high-pitched rhonchi and crepitations can be heard throughout the lungs. The infant should be admitted to hospital where intensive care is possible and artificial ventilation available if the dyspnoea worsens. The infants are nursed in extra oxygen. Antibiotics are often given as it is difficult to distinguish from pneumonia. Nasogastric tube feeding is likely to be needed for the very breathless infant, and careful attention has to be paid to fluid and calorie intake. The crisis lasts for 2–3 days only and then recovery gradually occurs. Up to half the infants diagnosed as having bronchiolitis subsequently develop recurrent wheezing (asthma).

156

Pneumonia

Bronchopneumonia

This is commonest in the younger child (Fig. 34), or in an older child who has some chronic condition, e.g. severe cerebral palsy. A wide variety of organisms can be responsible, and in the infant respiratory syncytial virus is the most important. It commonly follows bronchitis, measles and whooping cough.

Onset may be sudden or gradual, and fever is also variable. The specific features are rapid breathing and a

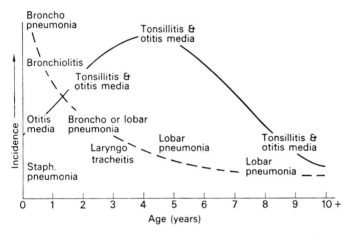

Fig. 34. The incidence of respiratory infections at different ages.

dry cough. Generalised crepitations and ronchi are present, and although chest X-ray shows small patches of consolidation it is unusual to detect them clinically. Cyanosis occurs in severe cases, and infants may develop cardiac failure.

Hospitalisation is usually needed. Oxygen and a broad-spectrum antibiotic are given. Gentle physiotherapy can help mobilise secretions.

Lobar pneumonia

157   This afflicts the 4–10-year-old child, and presents with

sudden illness and high fever. Pleuritic pain may be felt in the chest, causing the child to lean towards the affected side, or may be referred to the abdomen or neck. The child is sick, looks flushed, breathes fast with an expiratory grunt and is using the alae nasi. There may be a 'cold sore' (herpes simplex) on the lip. The respiratory rhythm may be reversed so that the pause comes after inspiration rather than expiration. There may be no cough. The clinical signs of consolidation may not be present at first but are usually apparent on X-ray, and repeated examination will usually reveal them. A transient pleural rub is common.

Lobar pneumonia is usually caused by the pneumococcus, and penicillin achieves dramatic improvement within 24 hours. Provided that conditions are reasonable, this is a safe and rewarding condition to treat at home. It is best to give the initial dose of penicillin by injection as an ill child is likely to vomit medicine. A hypnotic will ensure sleep for the child and, if there is a troublesome cough, a cough suppressant is given. Fluid intake is more important than food. Aspirin and tepid sponging help reduce fever.

If signs or symptoms are still present after a week, careful examination including chest X-ray should be repeated to exclude such complications as pleural effusion or lobar collapse.

Staphylococcal pneumonia

This is a severe form of pneumonia which affects infants, and children with fibrocystic disease. It is characterised by lung cysts on X-ray, and the sudden appearance of empyema or pneumothorax clinically. Lobar consolidation in an infant may be the first radiological sign. Prolonged treatment with an antibiotic effective against penicillin-resistant staphylococci is required.

Recurrent coughs and colds

Recurrent coughs and colds, sometimes with sore throat and earache, are very common in young children. Some babies and toddlers are catarrhal much of the time. If their colds spread to other members of the household and are worse in winter they are probably viral. If they are non-seasonal and do not spread they are probably of allergic origin. The first winter at school or nursery is frequently punctuated by upper respiratory infections.

Poor social circumstances predispose to catarrh. Some children will not blow their noses: some with severe nasal obstruction cannot. Cough persisting after pertussis may be due to lobar or segmental collapse. Night cough may be caused by a post-nasal drip (as with chronic sinus infection) or by mite sensitivity. Rarer causes of recurrent cough include cystic fibrosis, tuberculosis, and hiatus hernia.

If the cause cannot be eliminated, decongestants and cough suppressants will give symptomatic relief. The best healer is the passage of time.

Inhaled foreign bodies

Babies and toddlers are most at risk, for they tend to put everything into their mouths. Older children sometimes accidentally inhale objects during games or whilst stuffing their mouths too full of peanuts or sweets.

A foreign body may lodge at any level. At the time the child will cough, splutter or make choking noises but the episode is quickly forgotten and may not come out in the history without specific questioning. In the larynx an object is likely to cause a croupy cough and stridor. If it passes through the larynx it will lodge in a bronchus (right middle lobe or a lower lobe most often) and there will be no symptoms for a few days until infection, collapse or (less often) obstructive emphysema develop.

Whenever the possibility of a foreign body is suspected both anteroposterior and lateral X-rays of the neck and chest should be taken. Translucent objects may not show and the search may have to be continued by direct laryngoscopy and bronchoscopy, which would in any case be required to remove the object.

THE WHEEZY CHILD

Wheezing is an obstructive respiratory sound arising in the smaller branches of the bronchial tree; on auscultation rhonchi can be heard. They are most marked in expiration because the bronchial tree dilates in inspiration. The obstruction results from bronchospasm, mucosal oedema and secretions. Babies wheeze readily because their airways are small. Bronchospasm results from the release of spasmogens (e.g. histamine, serotonin) from the bronchial mucosal cells. Mucosal oedema may be of allergic or infective origin. The appearance of the nasal mucosa often reflects what is happening lower down the respiratory tract.

Recurrent wheezing is common in childhood. Some young children outgrow this phase of 'wheezy bronchitis', but others continue to have recurrent bouts of wheezing and eventually are diagnosed as having asthma.

Asthma is characterised by recurrent bouts of wheezing, breathlessness and cough due to intermittent, reversible obstruction of the peripheral airways. It tends to occur in response to a variety of stimuli, and most often in children with a personal or family history of allergy.

It is important to try to understand the underlying factors in each wheezy child if the best help is to be given. The principal factors are:

1 *Infection*. Bronchitis is common in young children and is often accompanied by wheezing (wheezy bronchitis). Wheezing is always a conspicuous feature of bronchiolitis. Infection is likely to be an important factor in those asthmatics who have most trouble in winter.

2 *Allergy*. Many asthmatics are sensitive to inhaled allergens, most commonly house-dust mite or grass pollens. Allergens can be best identified from the history (e.g. wheezing at night or in the pollen season) but skin tests and nasal provocation tests may be helpful. Skin tests are usually negative in children under 3 years and multiple reactions are common in older children. A family history of allergies is common.

3 *Atopy*. The atopic state is defined as an altered body response to foreign proteins. IgE is produced readily in response to common environmental antigens. It has a strong genetic basis and commonly manifests as asthma, hay fever, recurrent urticaria and/or eczema. In the family history atopy and allergy often overlap.

4 *Emotions*. Exceptionally, a severe emotional upset may precipitate a first attack of wheezing. Commonly, excitement or anxiety can precipitate attacks in known

asthmatics. Wheezing, especially if severe, causes anxiety and hence a bad attack may become self-perpetuating.

5 *Exertion*. Some asthmatics become wheezy on quite mild exertion, but further exercise may reverse the bronchoconstriction. Exercise-induced wheezing occurs most readily in a cold atmosphere.

6 *Atmosphere*. Dusty air, 'stuffy' rooms or changes in air temperature may all precipitate wheezing.

In young children upper respiratory tract infections appear to be the commonest precipitating factor, but as the child grows up others may become apparent—specific allergens, exercise, emotional upsets and changes of weather or environment.

Incidence

Up to 10% of infants have a tendency to wheeze in the first 2 years of life. Most grow out of it. About 3% of school children are considered to have asthma compared with a 1% incidence in adults, which suggests that many outgrow their asthma.

Clinical features

There is often a family history of asthma, eczema, urticaria or hay fever; and the child may have had, or develop, other hypersensitivity phenomena. Eczema is particularly common from 1 to 8 years of age, and hay fever in the schoolchild.

In the early years the child suffers from recurrent respiratory infections which persist longer than usual. Colds 'go to the chest', coughs persist, and the parents may notice wheezing. The wheezing may steadily worsen for a day or two before gradually improving. As the child becomes older the bouts become more clearly defined and more strikingly intermittent. The onset is sudden, and the child starts wheezing or coughing; breathlessness increases and with it fear. On examination the respiratory rate is increased and the child may be using the accessory muscles of respiration or pushing his hands against a table to force air out in expiration. The wheeze is mainly expiratory and on auscultation prolonged expiratory rhonchi are heard. Crepitations are variable.

Between attacks there are usually no symptoms or signs. Some children with frequent severe attacks develop hyperinflation, limited chest movement and hyperresonance. Useful indicators of severity are weight gain, days missed from school and peak expiratory flow rate. If no flowmeter is available, chest expansion can be measured with a tape measure.

Prevention

The aim is to reduce the frequency and severity of attacks and to give the child and family confidence that they can cope with attacks without disruption of home or school life. Precipitating factors should always be sought (Fig. 35). Although most schoolchildren produce positive skin reactions to pollens and house-dust mite, these tests have to be interpreted in the light of the clinical history. In all

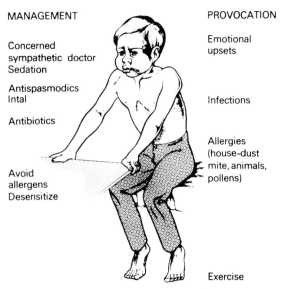

MANAGEMENT

Concerned
sympathetic doctor
Sedation

Antispasmodics
Intal

Antibiotics

Avoid
allergens
Desensitize

PROVOCATION

Emotional
upsets

Infections

Allergies
(house-dust
mite, animals,
pollens)

Exercise

Fig. 35. Precipitating factors in childhood asthma and possible solutions.

cases it is worth reducing the child's exposure to likely allergens such as bed house-dust mite and animals. The bedroom should be damp-dusted regularly, a plastic mattress cover used and pets banned from the bedroom. Emotional problems at home or school can often be· helped, but asthma generates its own emotional problems for the family. It can be a frightening condition for the child and family.

Disodium cromoglycate is a valuable prophylactic agent. It is inhaled as a powder from a spinhaler, usually four times daily. It is believed to interfere with the release of spasmogens from mast cells of the bronchial wall. Long-term therapy reduces the frequency of asthmatic attacks in a large proportion of children. The introduction of disodium cromoglycate and steroid aerosols has almost eliminated the necessity for oral corticosteroid therapy. It is difficult to persuade children under 5 to use inhalers effectively, but oral bronchodilator drugs may be effective.

Treatment of wheezing

The child should be up and about, leading as normal a life as possible, unless feeling really ill and feverish. A mild attack will often respond to oral antispasmodics such as theophylline derivatives, orciprenaline or (after the age of 18 months) salbutamol or terbutaline.

More severe attacks require to be stopped faster. Subcutaneous adrenaline or intravenous aminophylline act quickly, whilst aminophylline suppositories have the advantage that they can be administered by the parents. Pressurized aerosols containing sympathomimetic drugs are easily used by the patient, but over-use can be dangerous. Salbutamol aerosols are probably the safest, but strict instructions must be given and written down to limit the number of 'puffs' used. Salbutamol can be administered very effectively in hospital with a nebuliser. Whenever asthma appears to have been precipitated by infection, antibiotics are often given, though viruses are usually responsible.

Status asthmaticus describes a state in which severe bronchospasm has not responded to therapeutic measures, or has lasted for over 6 hours. It is a dangerous state, and the child should be admitted to hospital. In addition to the antispasmodics, sedatives and antibiotics previously mentioned, corticosteroids may be dramatically effective; it is unusual for them to be needed for more than 3 days. Oxygen is given to the very breathless or cyanosed child, and in extreme circumstances bronchial lavage may be needed to clear the obstructed airways of sticky secretions and intermittent positive pressure ventilation used. One of the curious features of status asthmaticus is that the act of admission to hospital sometimes stops the attack before any drugs have been given. This seems to be related more to the change in emotional atmosphere than to physical allergenic differences between home and hospital.

Asthma still causes a number of childhood deaths, usually when the attack has lasted several hours. Apart from mortality, the morbidity needs to be considered. Repeated attacks of asthma may lead to pulmonary complications, particularly emphysema and chronic bronchitis. Growth may be restricted, particularly if steroid treatment is needed. Educational and social problems may arise; some children who cannot manage at normal school are admitted to schools for the physically handicapped and delicate, and others to boarding school. This form of 'parentectomy' is reserved for the child who has intractable wheezing in the home environment. Family life can be completely overshadowed by the fact that one child has asthma. This should be rare; asthma is a challenge which the doctor can help the family to overcome.

Further reading

Godfrey S. *Your Child with Asthma—Some Advice for Parents and Others*, Heinemann.
Williams H. E. & Phelan P. D. *Respiratory Illness in Children*, Blackwell Scientific Publications.

Chapter 12

The Alimentary Tract

Like most childhood illness, alimentary tract disorders are usually acute and infective. These are most serious in infancy, when fluid and electrolyte balance can become dangerously disturbed within a matter of hours and cause death or brain damage if not recognized and treated. Intestinal obstructions are also important and may be of congenital origin or acquired. Less common, but equally important, are malabsorption states including coeliac disease and cystic fibrosis. In childhood, peptic ulcers, ulcerative colitis and Crohn's disease are uncommon, and neoplasm very rare.

SYMPTOMS AND SIGNS OF ALIMENTARY DISORDERS

The principal symptoms of acute alimentary disease are vomiting, diarrhoea and abdominal pain; of chronic disease, failure to thrive and diarrhoea. Constipation is, of course, a feature of acute intestinal obstruction, but chronic constipation and recurrent abdominal pain are not commonly due to alimentary tract disease. Abdominal distension is a feature of some acute and some chronic disorders.

It is very common for babies to bring up a small amount of food when breaking wind after a feed. This is possetting, a normal process that may be confused with vomiting by an inexperienced mother. Possetting is not accompanied by other symptoms, the baby is happy and gains weight well. Significant vomiting (Table 9) will be accompanied by weight loss, or at least by inadequate weight gain. Forceful (projectile) vomiting suggests high intestinal obstruction.

Haematemesis is not a common symptom in childhood.

Table 9. Causes of vomiting

1. Feeding errors
   (a) In infants, too much food, too little food, the wrong kind of food, or faulty feeding technique
   (b) In older children, dietetic indiscretions
2. Infections
   (a) Gastritis (with or without enteritis)
   (b) Parenteral infections (e.g. tonsillitis, meningitis)
   (c) Acute appendicitis
3. Mechanical causes
   (a) Intestinal obstruction, congenital or acquired
   (b) Hiatus hernia: lax oesophagus
4. Raised intracranial pressure
   (a) Meningitis: encephalitis
   (b) Space-occupying lesions (tumour, abscess, haematoma)
5. Metabolic disorders
   (a) Inborn errors of metabolism
   (b) Adrenal insufficiency
   (c) Ketosis; uraemia
   (d) Intolerance of, or allergy to, food components (e.g. gluten, lactose)
6. Psychological problems
   (a) Periodic syndrome ('cyclical vomiting'): migraine
   (b) Rumination
7. Miscellaneous
   (a) Travel sickness
   (b) Poisoning

Small amounts of fresh or altered blood in the vomitus are seen if blood from the nose or throat has been swallowed, with gastritis and oesophagitis. Massive haematemesis may also result from swallowed blood (e.g. after tonsillectomy), oesophageal or gastric varices or peptic ulcer. If the history raises the possibility of recent haematemesis but is not conclusive, check the stools for occult blood.

In the same way, the existence of diarrhoea or constipation should not be accepted without detailed enquiry. The number and consistency of stools passed by children, especially infants, is very variable and is influenced by diet. Breast-fed babies pass loose, bright yellow, odourless stools, usually three or four times a day but often after every feed and sometimes as infrequently as once a week. Bottle-fed babies pass paler, firmer, more acid stools which smell. If fed on evaporated milk, the consistency and frequency may be similar to that of a breast-fed baby: if fed on dried milk, the stools are usually formed and may be quite hard, causing the baby to strain when defaecating. Unless this straining causes pain or rectal bleeding, or the bowels are being opened less than once a day, this should not be called constipation. Many toddlers and some older children (and some adults) continue to have 3 or 4 bowel actions a day, after meals ('toddler diarrhoea'). If the stool consistency and weight gain are satisfactory, this is not abnormal. Frequent stools are often associated with a rapid transit time, and undigested food may be recognised in the stool within a few hours of being eaten (our personal best was carrots at 20 minutes). Chronic constipation (p. 124) may lead to faecal impaction and soiling, which may be mistakenly interpreted as diarrhoea. The principal causes of diarrhoea are shown in Table 10.

Abdominal pain is an important symptom but does not necessarily indicate abdominal disease. Acute central abdominal pain and vomiting are, for example, common symptoms of tonsillitis in young children. Recurrent abdominal pain may be a symptom of emotional stress. From about the age of 2 years children can indicate the site of a pain. In infants, abdominal pain may be inferred from spasms of crying, restlessness and drawing up the knees. It is a very common symptom throughout childhood and is usually of no serious significance. The presence of vomiting, bowel disturbance or fever in

Table 10. Causes of diarrhoea

1. Feeding errors
   (a) In infants, too much food, too little or the wrong kind
   (b) In older children, dietetic indiscretion
2. Inflammatory lesions
   (a) Enteritis, including dysentery
   (b) Ulcerative colitis: Crohn's disease
   (c) Giardiasis (lambliasis)
   (d) Parenteral infections
3. Malabsorption states
   (a) Steatorrhoea (coeliac disease: cystic fibrosis)
   (b) Disaccharide intolerance
   (c) Protein-losing enteropathy

association with abdominal pain should prompt a more detailed appraisal, with re-examination after a few hours.

Abdominal distension can be difficult to assess because of the very great normal variation. Fat babies appear to have bigger tummies than thin, muscular babies. Toddlers are normally rather pot-bellied in comparison with older children and coloured children in comparison with white. The mother will usually be able to say whether the abdomen is swollen.

It is important to recognize dehydration and wasting, especially in infants. Clinical dehydration results from inadequate fluid intake (which is not common) or excessive loss by vomiting, diarrhoea or polyuria. The combination of diarrhoea and vomiting, which is inevitably accompanied by inadequate intake, leads to losses of fluid and electrolytes. This is seen in its most dramatic form in infantile gastroenteritis ('D and V'). The anterior fontanelle and the eyes become sunken, the skin loses its normal elasticity, the infant has an anxious look, a persistent cry and is restless. If the condition progresses, the baby becomes quiet and still, with sunken abdomen and signs of peripheral circulatory failure. In the older child, the lips and tongue become dry, and the eyes a little sunken. After infancy, vomiting rapidly leads to ketosis which is recognized by the smell of the breath and acidotic beathing. Dehydration at any age, if it results from vomiting and/or diarrhoea, will lead to a reduced urinary output: measurement of urine output is therefore helpful when practicable.

Examination of the abdomen

Examination of the abdomen in children requires patience, gentleness and a warm hand. It is helpful for the doctor to get down to the same level as the child by sitting or kneeling, unless the child is on a high bed or couch. This not only makes palpation more satisfactory, it makes conversation easier and the apprehensive child is saved from being towered over. As with older patients, palpation should at first be very gentle, especially if some painful condition is suspected. The right side of the abdomen is sometimes more easily felt from the left side of the patient, either by going round the other side of the cot or by turning the child head to toes. Thus, the liver and the right kidney may be more easily felt. In suspected pyloric stenosis, examination must always be from the left side of the infant.

The liver is normally palpable in infants and toddlers. In babies, the edge is usually about 2 cm below the costal margin. A palpable spleen tip is not necessarily abnormal. The kidneys can usually be felt, the right more easily than the left, if the abdomen is reasonably thin and well relaxed. Faecal masses are commonly felt in the line of the colon. Small bowel peristalsis may be visible if the abdominal wall is very thin, as in small pre-term babies and children with wasting diseases. Remember to examine hernial orifices.

Rectal examination is rarely omitted by surgeons and often forgotten by physicians. It may be disturbing to young or nervous children, and the decision whether or not to make a rectal examination depends upon what is likely to be learned from it. The doctor is unlikely to detect localised tenderness if the child is crying before he starts. The little finger should be used for rectal examination in infants, the index finger in older children.

Examination of a stool, which should be as fresh as possible, is often informative. The colour, consistency and smell are noted; the presence of blood or mucus; and the pH (paper strip tests) and sugar (clinitest tablet). Microscopy combined with the use of a fat stain will show fat globules and undigested meat fibres in malabsorption states.

The teeth

The ages of usual appearance of the teeth are listed in Appendix 4. There is considerable normal variation in the time of eruption of teeth which may lead to unnecessary worry. The first teeth are sometimes apparent at birth, or no teeth may be cut until after the first birthday. Such extreme variations are usually physiological. Preventive dental health is important for all children, especially the handicapped. An adequate fluoride intake halves dental decay. Sweets encourage decay, and doctors should avoid prescribing sucrose-containing syrups for long-term use.

Regular tooth-cleaning and dental supervision should be encouraged.

It is good practice for the doctor to include the teeth in his examination of the mouth. It gives an opportunity for either congratulation or health education, and occasionally an unexpected alveolar abscess is found to explain a persistent fever or ill health.

Stomatitis

In infancy, stomatitis is usually due to *Candida albicans* (monilia; thrush). This may develop in any baby whose feeds, bottles, teats or dummy have not been adequately sterilized; in babies who have been given broad-spectrum antibiotics, even for a few days only; and in emaciated and very ill infants. It appears as tiny white flecks inside the cheeks, on the tongue and on the roof of the mouth. The only possible source of diagnostic confusion is milk curds which are usually larger than thrush lesions, and can easily be detached with a spatula. *Candida albicans* will be cultured in large numbers from a swab (but it should be noted that this organism can often be cultured from the mouths or throats of healthy children). Treatment is aimed first at the cause (correction of faulty sterilization techniques or review of antibiotic policy) and second at elimination of the organism by the local application of nystatin or (in nystatin-resistant cases) amphotericin B. It is important to continue local application for a few days after apparent cure, otherwise recurrence is likely.

Candida albicans may also infect the skin of the napkin area (p. 204) and it may cause systemic infection in children with immunological deficiencies or debilitating diseases.

In older children, stomatitis is usually due to a first infection with herpesvirus hominis Type I. *Herpetic stomatitis* is most common in toddlers, and the lesions are most marked on the lips and tongue. There are vesicles, ulcers and scabs and the condition is painful. The gums are inflamed. There is cervical adenitis. Because of the pain the child will not eat and is often reluctant even to drink. There is general misery, listlessness and a low-grade fever. The condition is self-limiting: the discomfort eases after a few days, and the lesions have healed in 2 weeks. Admission to hospital may be necessary to maintain fluid intake. Local applications are of doubtful value. Antibiotics should be avoided because they encourage super-added infection with *Candida albicans*.

Herpangina is the term given to upper respiratory infections associated with ulcers which are confined to the posterior pharynx and fauces. The usual causes are viruses of the Coxsackie A group. In some children the ulcers are associated with vesicles on the hands, feet and buttocks—'Hand, foot and mouth disease'.

HERNIAS

Hernias in children may involve the umbilicus, the diaphragm, the inguinal or femoral regions. They differ in some important ways from the hernias of adults.

Umbilical hernia

This is common and harmless. There is a small, sharply defined, circular defect in the centre of the umbilicus through which protrudes a small loop of bowel. Umbilical hernia is always easily reducible and virtually never strangulates. Spontaneous cure is usual before the first birthday. Treatment is not required although adhesive strapping may support the mother's morale. Babies with umbilical hernia may cry (as may babies without hernias) but the hernia should not be regarded as the cause of the crying. In para-umbilical hernia, the orifice is usually immediately above the centre of the umbilicus. This may not heal spontaneously, and surgical repair will be required before the child starts school. Umbilical hernia is an almost constant feature of cretinism, in which the hernia may be quite large. It heals when the cretinism is treated with thyroxin.

Diaphragmatic hernia

The most serious type of diaphragmatic hernia causes difficulties from the moment of birth and results from the failure of one or other leaf of the diaphragm (rarely both) to develop. It is more common on the left side. The lung on the side of the hernia is usually grossly underdeveloped.

The hemithorax contains abdominal viscera, the heart is displaced to the opposite side, and the contralateral lung is compressed by the mediastinum. There is therefore grave respiratory difficulty from the moment of birth. If the hernia is left-sided, examination reveals the heart beat on the right side of the chest; if on the right, the apex beat is in the left axilla. Percussion note and air entry may be abnormal, but it is unusual to hear bowel sounds except with small hernias that gradually develop over a few days. A chest radiograph makes the diagnosis clear. Early intubation and positive pressure insufflation are usually necessary to maintain life until surgical repair can be undertaken.

Hiatus hernia associated with congenital short oesophagus is more common but less serious. It presents with vomiting in early infancy, sometimes in the neonatal period. There may be a small amount of fresh or altered blood in the vomitus. The vomiting is not projectile, and weight gain is usually maintained. The diagnosis may be confirmed radiologically by giving a contrast meal. A small knuckle of stomach can be demonstrated above the diaphragm. In the head-down position oesophageal reflux can be demonstrated, and reflux can occur without hiatus hernia. Reflux with or without hernia is usually more of a nuisance than a worry, and conservative management is indicated. This consists of nursing the baby in the sitting position in a baby seat, thickening milk feeds and introducing solid foods as early as possible. Remission of symptoms can be anticipated towards the end of the first year of life. Exceptionally, a large hiatus hernia causes copious vomiting and weight loss. Surgical repair is required.

Inguinal hernia

This is common in boys, rare in girls. It is often bilateral. A big hernia will form a large swelling in the scrotum, which can be reduced quite easily if the baby is quiet. A small hernia will cause a swelling in the groin which may only be visible intermittently. The smaller the hernia, the more liable it is to strangulate. The doctor should therefore be more concerned about the hernia he cannot see than the one he can. In either case, the danger is present and spontaneous cure is not to be anticipated. Surgical repair should be undertaken at the first convenient moment.

INTESTINAL OBSTRUCTION

Intestinal obstruction may be present at birth, usually as a consequence of malformations of the alimentary tract, or may develop at any age thereafter. The cardinal symptoms are vomiting, abdominal distension, constipation, and (in children old enough to make their feelings clear) pain. Vomiting will lead to fluid and electrolyte loss with clinical signs of dehydration, and later to circulatory failure. Successful treatment therefore depends upon early diagnosis, adequate pre-operative correction of fluid and electrolyte loss, and skilled surgery and anaesthesia.

1 In the newborn

The level of the obstruction in the newborn may be anywhere from the oesophagus to the anus. Because swallowing by the fetus is one of the normal routes of disposal of amniotic fluid, obstruction may lead to accumulation of excess fluid (polyhydramnios) before birth, thus providing a diagnostic clue. The higher the level of obstruction, the more likely is this to occur. It is therefore common with oesophageal atresia but rare with rectal atresia. (Stenosis indicates narrowing of a passage: atresia indicates complete obstruction.) *Oesophageal atresia* is usually associated with tracheo-oesophageal fistula (Fig. 36) so that the bowel is soon filled with air via the fistula. In the absence of a fistula, the bowel remains airless and the abdomen sunken. Because swallowing is impossible, mucus tends to accumulate in the pharynx, and the infant after birth needs frequent aspiration of secretions. True vomiting is impossible, as food cannot reach the stomach, but if feeding is attempted, there will be immediate regurgitation and inhalation of feeds, with choking and cyanosis. Milk in the lungs causes severe pneumonia, and diagnosis should be made before feeding. If there has been polyhydramnios, or if suspicions are aroused by excess secretions, a naso-gastric tube should

Fig. 36. Tracheo-oesophageal fistula before and after surgical correction.

be passed to demonstrate patency of the oesophagus. If this proves impossible, radiography after the careful instillation of a few millilitres of contrast medium into the oesophageal pouch will confirm the diagnosis and demonstrate the level of the obstruction. Early diagnosis and skilled surgery offer the best chance of cure, but there are other severe defects in about half the cases. Oesophageal and rectal atresia sometimes occur in the same baby.

Atresias at lower levels will cause vomiting and distension. If the obstruction is high, vomiting will be early. The vomit will contain bile because the obstruction is usually below the ampulla of Vater. Distension will be mainly epigastric. If the obstruction is lower, the vomiting will start a little later and the distension will be more generalised. *Duodenal atresia* and stenosis are particularly common in mongols. *Rectal atresia* is usually associated with fistula between the rectum and some part of the genito-urinary tract. An infant with low, complete obstruction cannot pass meconium, but small quantities may be passed by those with high obstruction. In *Hirschsprung's disease*, obstruction is incomplete and is due to a narrow, aganglionic segment of bowel, most commonly in the recto-sigmoid region. *Meconium ileus* is a manifestation of cystic fibrosis (p. 181). In *malrotation*, the bowel has become twisted at the time of reduction of the normal umbilical hernia of embryonic life and obstruction results from peritoneal bands. There are many other causes of congenital obstruction, and often the precise anatomical diagnosis can only be made at operation. The site of obstruction can often be deduced from the distribution of intestinal gas seen on a straight radiograph taken with the baby vertical. If there is imperforate anus or low rectal atresia, a radiograph is taken with the baby inverted and a metal marker over the anal dimple: the distance from the terminal gas shadow to the marker indicates the depth at which the bowel ends.

In *exomphalos* (omphalocele) the temporary umbilical hernia of normal embryonic development has become permanent, and the baby is born with a variable amount of bowel and other abdominal viscera protruding from the umbilicus. If the viscera are enclosed in a membrane, conservative measures sometimes give good results, but surgical repair is usually undertaken and is imperative if there is no covering membrane. The term *gastroschisis* describes a more severe and serious congenital defect of the abdominal wall.

2 At later ages

Intestinal obstruction at later ages may be caused by intussusception, pyloric stenosis, volvulus, strangulated inguinal hernia or other rarer causes. *Intussusception* occurs most commonly in infancy. It has been suggested that the change to a mixed diet leads to a change in intestinal flora and that this causes hypertrophy of Peyer's patches, one of which may form the apex of an intussusception. There is also evidence to suggest that viral infections of the bowel may play a role in causation. The infant cries intermittently with colicky abdominal pain, and between attacks is quiet and pale. The spasms become more frequent and more severe, red blood may be passed with a rather loose stool ('red-currant jelly'), and distension and vomiting soon develop. Gentle palpation, preferably while the infant is asleep between attacks of pain, will often reveal a firm, sausage-shaped mass lying somewhere in the line of the colon, often in the upper right quadrant. Rarely, the apex may be felt on rectal examination. In cases of diagnostic difficulty, a contrast enema, given with care, may show the intussusception, and on occasion may cause its reduction. However, the treatment of choice is reduction at open operation, after correction of fluid and electrolyte balance, with resection of any gangrenous bowel.

Pyloric stenosis

Congenital pyloric stenosis is a relatively common condition, the cause of which is still unknown. The marked preponderance in males (about sevenfold), the increased incidence in co-twins, and in close relatives, suggest that there is a genetic contribution to the disorder. On the other hand, it is rarely found in stillborn babies, or babies dying within a few days of birth, and it is therefore arguable whether it should be called 'congenital'. The pathology is a hypertrophy of the circular muscle of the pylorus which leads to progressive obstruction. The onset of symptoms is usually gradual, beginning in the second or third week of life, though occasionally much later. Vomiting is initially slight and intermittent but becomes more frequent, more copious and more forceful (projectile vomiting). Weight gain, which has usually been satisfactory before the onset of symptoms, falls off, eventually stops, and is followed by weight loss. The motions become more and more constipated. Appetite remains ravenous, but if diagnosis is delayed wasting and dehydration follow (Fig. 37). Pyloric stenosis is diagnosed by watching the infant feed, a procedure which may take half an hour. A mass may be felt in the pyloric region before the feed begins, but is often more evident after the feed has been vomited. It is the shape and size of a large olive, very firm, and may be felt contracting intermittently. As the stomach fills, waves of peristalsis become visible, crossing the epigastrium from left to right. Gastric peristalsis tends to become more and more marked until the infant vomits, when the vomitus may shoot out several feet. If there is diagnostic difficulty, a contrast meal will show a distended stomach, and a narrow, elongated pyloric canal. The treatment of choice is surgical, the pyloric

Worried hungry expression

Projectile vomiting after a feed

Palpable pyloric mass during feed, and visible peristalsis

Constipated

Thin, with signs of weight loss

7 boys : 1 girl age 1-10 weeks

Fig. 37. Pyloric stenosis.

muscle being divided along its entire length until the mucosa bulges up into the incision (Ramstedt's* operation). Success depends upon adequate preoperative preparation, skilled surgery and anaesthesia, and careful post-operative management. If for any reason surgical treatment cannot be carried out, the condition can be treated medically by giving antispasmodics (atropine methyl nitrate or scopolamine methyl nitrate) shortly before each feed. Medical treatment has to be continued for weeks or months, after which the condition resolves. It is therefore tedious, and weight gain may remain unsatisfactory.

177   * Ramstedt and Rammstedt are both correct: he used both.

INFECTIVE DIARRHOEA

Acute, infective diarrhoea is common, it spreads rapidly through a closed community like a home or a hospital ward, and it is potentially lethal, especially in the very young. The cause may be viral or bacterial, and a similar illness may result from the ingestion of bacterial exotoxins or chemical poisons. Rotaviruses are common pathogens throughout childhood. Bacterial infections in infants are often due to pathogenic *E. coli*: their pathogenicity depends more on their ability to produce enterotoxins than on their serotype. In older children, infections with Salmonella and Shigella organisms predominate.

In gastroenteritis diarrhoea and vomiting (D and V) quickly upset fluid and electrolyte balance. Dehydration causes fretfulness, sunken eyes and fontanelle, and a dry, inelastic skin. Urine output falls: blood urea rises. In some infants water is lost more rapidly than electrolytes causing a rise in serum sodium above 150 mmol/l (*hypernatraemic dehydration*), a condition which may be difficult to diagnose and to treat. In the very young there may be fever and leucocytosis, suggesting systemic spread of the infection. In these infants, the administration of appropriate antibiotics is probably helpful. In older children with Salmonella and Shigella infections, antibiotics may delay clearing of the pathogens from the bowel. The basis of treatment is the correction and maintenance of fluid and electrolyte balance. Mild cases may be treated at home by giving small volumes of water at frequent intervals for 24 hours followed by gradual re-introduction of milk. Moderate and severe cases require an intravenous drip until oral fluids can be retained, and strict barrier nursing to prevent the spread of infection to others.

MALABSORPTION STATES

In children, malabsorption equates closely with steatorrhoea. There are conditions in which the digestion and absorption of sugars is abnormal, and protein-losing enteropathy occurs very rarely, but where fatty diarrhoea occurs much more frequently. Again, there are many possible causes of fatty diarrhoea, but in practice it usually turns out to be due to either coeliac disease or cystic fibrosis of the pancreas. In both conditions the stools are offensive, pale and bulky as well as frequent, and sometimes the mother reports difficulty in flushing them down the toilet because of their tendency to float. Weight gain is unsatisfactory, or there may be frank weight loss with muscle wasting. This contrasts with the big abdomen which is due predominantly to gaseous distension of the bowel.

Coeliac disease

Coeliac disease is the result of a sensitivity to the gluten fraction of wheat, rye or other cereals. Therefore symptoms are not to be expected before the introduction of cereals into the diet. There is evidence to suggest that earlier introduction of cereals leads to an increased incidence of coeliac disease. (Infants do not need cereals before 4 months of age.) In addition to the fatty diarrhoea, wasting and abdominal distension described above, the appetite is usually very poor and the child is miserable. Many of the children have a fair complexion and long eyelashes (Fig. 38 and cover picture). The liver is often impalpable. Sometimes the disease begins acutely, and in these children vomiting may be more conspicuous than diarrhoea: indeed, the combination of vomiting and abdominal distension may suggest intestinal obstruction.

There is an enormous range of investigations to which the child suspected of having coeliac disease may be subjected. The diagnosis should not be made without jejunal biopsy, which shows sub-total villous atrophy (a flat appearance) when examined with a dissecting microscope. Therefore it is arguable that no other test is necessary. However, there are many children in whom the diagnosis is more of a possibility than a probability, and in such cases alternative tests may be accepted as adequate to exclude the diagnosis. A xylose absorption test, in which a single estimation of blood xylose is made one hour after a loading dose of oral xylose, seems more informative in children than the conventional xylose tolerance test. A small bowel contrast meal may also be helpful.

Fair complexion

Long eyelashes

Miserable, poor appetite

+ fatty diarrhoea and vomiting Impalpable liver

Abdominal distension

Muscle wasting

Fig. 38. Coeliac disease.

Treatment consists of exclusion of wheat and rye gluten, and others if necessary. There is usually a rapid and dramatic effect on appetite and temperament, followed by a good weight gain, but some children do not show improvement until they have been on their diet for 3 or 4 weeks. A few children with coeliac disease also have a temporary intolerance of lactose and do not improve until this has also been eliminated from the diet. Iron-deficiency anaemia is common (megaloblastic anaemia rare), and the rapid growth that follows treatment may precipitate rickets. Iron and vitamin supplements are therefore indicated in the early stages of treatment. Although it is often possible for a coeliac child to return to a normal diet in later childhood without a recurrence of diarrhoea, growth may suffer and there is a significant incidence of small bowel lymphoma in adult coeliacs. Strict dietary control for life is therefore advisable.

Gluten intolerance in the first 2 years of life is sometimes a temporary phenomenon. Re-evaluation and repeat biopsy after gluten challenge is often needed to clarify diagnosis.

Cystic fibrosis (fibrocystic disease of the pancreas)

Cystic fibrosis is a serious disease which affects about one child in every 2–3000 amongst white races. In this ethnic group it is the commonest disease caused by an autosomal recessive gene, about 1 person in 23 carrying the gene. The fundamental defect has not yet been determined, but concerns transport across cell membranes. The symptoms of the disease, though varied, are largely attributable to the secretion of abnormally viscid mucus. The most helpful laboratory test demonstrates increased concentrations of sodium and chloride in sweat, saliva and other body secretions.

Cystic fibrosis may present clinically:
1 as intestinal obstruction in the newborn;
2 as failure to thrive with fatty diarrhoea, or
3 with recurrent respiratory infections.

In the newborn baby, the meconium may be so glutinous because of the viscid mucus in it that normal peristaltic waves cannot shift it (meconium ileus). Small amounts of meconium may be passed: generalized abdominal distension develops over 24–48 hours, and vomiting develops at the same time. An X-ray of the erect abdomen shows evidence of obstruction. At operation there is often obstruction at several sites, and clearing the viscid meconium may be very difficult. The bowel may have to be opened in several places, and washouts with mucolytic agents may be helpful. Unfortunately, even if the obstruction is overcome, the underlying disease remains. Prolapse of the rectum may occur in newborns with cystic fibrosis.

If affected infants pass through the neonatal period without illness, they are likely to present later in infancy because of offensive diarrhoea, poor weight gain, respiratory infections, or combinations of these symptoms. Malabsorption is chiefly due to blockage of the pancreatic ducts by viscid secretions and consequent deficiency of pancreatic enzymes. The diarrhoea may start any time from birth, and it is not related to changes in diet. Distension and weight loss resemble those seen in coeliac disease, but the appetite often remains good and the temperament less miserable than in coeliac disease (Fig. 39). Recurrent bronchitis and pneumonia (especially

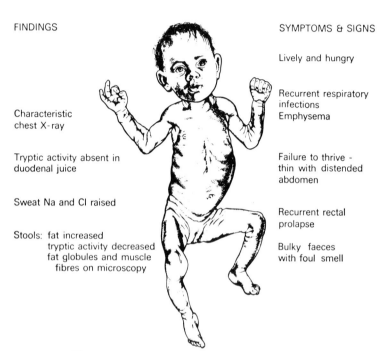

FINDINGS

Characteristic
chest X-ray

Tryptic activity absent in
duodenal juice

Sweat Na and Cl raised

Stools: fat increased
tryptic activity decreased
fat globules and muscle
fibres on microscopy

SYMPTOMS & SIGNS

Lively and hungry

Recurrent respiratory
infections
Emphysema

Failure to thrive -
thin with distended
abdomen

Recurrent rectal
prolapse

Bulky faeces
with foul smell

Fig. 39. Cystic fibrosis.

staphylococcal) may begin in infancy or may be delayed for several years. A few children suffer more from sinusitis and nasal polyposis than from chest infections.

Laboratory diagnosis rests chiefly on the demonstration of raised sodium and chloride levels (over 60 mmol/l in the sweat). Localized sweating is induced by iontophoresis with pilocarpine, and either the sweat is tested in situ by application of an appropriate electrode, or it is absorbed onto filter paper and analysed chemically. The test is not reliable in very young babies, but thereafter is remarkably specific. (Some mothers notice that the baby tastes salty when kissed.)

182

Treatment of the pancreatic disorder is relatively simple and consists in the provision of enzymes in powder or tablet form to be taken with food, together with supplements of iron and fat-soluble vitamins initially. Oral aluminium hydroxide improves the smell of the stools. If malabsorption is severe, synthetic diets incorporating medium-chain triglycerides may be helpful, but are unpalatable.

The respiratory problems tend to become slowly but progressively worse leading to extensive bronchiectasis and cor pulmonale. The main aim of therapy is therefore the prevention of chest infections, and depends upon physiotherapy and chemotherapy. The parents are taught to carry out postural drainage daily. Chemoprophylaxis, using antibiotics systemically or by inhalation, is used continuously or intermittently, according to circumstances. Saline inhalation may liquefy viscid secretions. In addition to direct treatment of the disease, progressive disability may demand education at a school for the physically handicapped; the parents require genetic counselling; and the family needs continuing support through a long, demanding, and at times distressing illness.

Disaccharide intolerance

Intolerance of disaccharides, notably lactose, may occur:
1   As a temporary complication of steatorrhoea in coeliac disease or cystic fibrosis.
2   As a temporary complication of gastroenteritis (or other infections).
3   Permanently, as a result of deficiency of lactase, usually genetically determined.

The condition causes a fermentative diarrhoea. It is diagnosed by demonstrating disaccharides in the stools, which are acid; deficiency of disaccharidases in jejunal biopsy specimens; and a good clinical response to the exclusion of the offending sugar. If the intolerance is temporary, lactose may be cautiously reintroduced once recovery from the underlying cause is complete.

Note: Although children with galactosaemia (p. 250) cannot tolerate lactose, the lesion is not in the alimentary tract and the disease is not usually classified as an intolerance.

OTHER ALIMENTARY DISORDERS

Food allergy

True allergy to foods is not common but does happen. The food proteins most often associated with allergy are cow's milk albumin and the proteins of fish, shellfish and some fruits (strawberries are most notorious). Symptoms of food allergy include vomiting, diarrhoea and abdominal pain; urticarial, erythematous or eczematous rashes; and exceptionally acute anaphylactic symptoms. The diagnosis is supported by appropriate skin tests and confirmed by relief of symptoms when the offending food is excluded, and recurrence when it is re-introduced. Oral disodium cromoglycate may be helpful.

Ulcerative colitis and Crohn's disease

Neither of these conditions is common in childhood, and they do not differ in essentials from the adult pattern. Ulcerative colitis most commonly presents with chronic or recurrent bloody diarrhoea with weight loss. Crohn's disease (regional ileitis) most commonly presents with obstructive symptoms. In the diagnosis of both conditions barium enema, sigmoidoscopy and colon biopsy are helpful. In neither disease is the cause understood, so treatment is empirical and not very satisfactory. Physicians modify the diet and prescribe sulphasalazine and steroids; surgeons resect the offending part; neither lays extravagant claims to success.

Acute abdominal pain

Appendicitis occurs at all ages but is uncommon under the age of 2. The most constant features are pain, vomiting, fever and a coated tongue. The diagnosis is usually made on the basis of localized tenderness. With appendix abscess, the history is longer and there is a palpable, tender mass. Diagnostic difficulties may be caused by an appendix in an unusual position, and by other conditions presenting with acute abdominal pain and vomiting. Once an inflamed appendix perforates and peritonitis supervenes, the prognosis becomes worse. If in doubt 'look and see' is wiser than 'wait and see'.

Toddlers with tonsillitis often complain of pain in the abdomen and not in the throat. Their abdominal tenderness is usually generalized or central, but may be maximal in the right iliac fossa. (Warning: tonsillitis and appendicitis can occur together.)

In acute pyelonephritis the tenderness is usually in the loins. Microscopy of the urine gives the diagnosis.

In right lower lobe pneumonia there may be referred pain and tenderness in the right iliac fossa. The respiratory rate will be raised, there are usually abnormal signs in the chest, and a chest X-ray is helpful.

Mesenteric adenitis is most confidently diagnosed at laparotomy, when enlarged, inflamed glands and normal appendix are found. The condition may be suspected clinically if the child is more tender than ill and if enlarged glands can be felt.

Giardiasis and worms

Giardia lamblia is a protozoon which commonly inhabits the alimentary canals of children without disturbing their health. Occasionally it causes disease, and this usually takes the form of chronic diarrhoea with semiformed, khaki-coloured stools and very little constitutional upset. Rarely, infection is associated with steatorrhoea and a clinical picture resembling coeliac disease. The cysts may be identified in the stools, although their presence does not establish that they are causing disease. Isolation of organisms from duodenal aspirate is more significant. Treatment is with mepacrine or metronidazole.

Intestinal worms are now seen far less often than they used to be. *Threadworms* (*Enterobius vermicularis*) are relatively common. They cause no symptoms apart from peri-anal itching which may disturb sleep. Diagnosis is made by seeing the worms on the peri-anal skin or stool, or by demonstrating ova from the peri-anal region, best achieved by the use of cellophane swabs or Sellotape. Piperazine is the drug of choice, often given as a single dose combined with standardized senna. Apparent failure is usually due to re-infection. Success is then often achieved by treating the whole family, including parents.

The *roundworm* (*Ascaris lumbricoides*) is uncommon. There are usually no symptoms before a worm is passed with the stools. Piperazine is the drug of choice. *Tapeworms* (*Taenia saginata* and *T. solium*) are now exceedingly rare because of high standards of butchering and domestic cooking. They present with the passage of segments. Treatment may be difficult. Niclosamide is probably the drug of choice.

Table 11. Causes of rectal bleeding

Site	Condition	Clinical picture
Ileum	Intussusception	Colicky pain: red-current jelly stool: palpable mass
	Bleeding Meckel's diverticulum	Intermittent abdominal pain and bleeding (red or melaena)
Colon	Dysentery (Shigella, Salmonella)	Acute mucoid diarrhoea and pain
	Ulcerative colitis	Mucoid diarrhoea; onset sometimes acute
	Intussusception	
Rectum	Polyp	Recurrent bleeding: no pain
	Prolapse	Prolapse visible
Anus	Fissure	On defaecation, much pain and little blood
	Constipation	

Rectal bleeding

Blood in the stools is always an alarming symptom, although the cause is often trivial. Bleeding from the duodenum or above will usually cause melaena, although copious bleeding (e.g. swallowed blood after epistaxis or tonsillectomy) may cause red blood to appear with the stool. Blood from the ileum or colon is freely mixed with faecal matter: that from the rectum or anus is only on the surface of the stool. If rectal bleeding is associated with painful defaecation, the likely cause is an anal fissure. If a fissure is seen, rectal examination would be very painful and should be avoided.

Many of the important causes of rectal bleeding in adults (e.g. piles, rectal carcinoma) do not occur in children. The main causes in childhood are shown in Table 11.

Meckel's diverticulum often contains gastric mucosa which may ulcerate and bleed, causing rectal bleeding and anaemia. Radioactive technetium is selectively taken up by gastric mucosa and this provides the basis for an elegant diagnostic test.

Further reading

Anderson C.M. & Burke V. *Paediatric Gastroenterology*, Black-well Scientific Publications.

Walker-Smith J. *Diseases of the Small Intestine in Childhood*, Pitman Medical.

Chapter 13

The Skeletal System

STRUCTURAL VARIATION AND CONGENITAL ABNORMALITIES

The normal flat-footed baby becomes a bow-legged toddler and then a knock-kneed primary school child before growing into a graceful adolescent (Fig. 40). Therefore one has to decide whether the source of the parents concern is normal physiological variation or something requiring further investigation and treatment.

The child should be examined standing and lying in order to detect abnormality of posture, and to check for equal size and length of the limbs. The child should be observed walking or running, and the shoes examined for abnormal wear.

Flat feet

At birth the feet look flat. When children start to stand, at the end of the first year, the feet still look flat because there is a large pad of fat on the soles. The child starts to walk on a wide base with the feet everted and the tibiae externally rotated, and the feet still look flat. By the 3rd year the eversion and external rotation have diminished and the feet begin to appear to have a normal plantar arch.

Bow legs (genu varum)

Bow legs are commonest from 0–2 years. The knees may be 5 cm apart when the feet are together; the toes point medially (Fig. 41). If the degree of bowing is gross, rickets should be excluded.

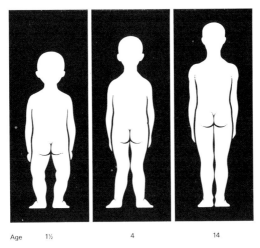

Age   1½   4   14

Fig. 40. Normal variation of legs with age.

Knock knees (genu valgum)

This is most apparent at 3–4 years of age. When the knees are together the medial malleoli may be up to 5 cm apart. In obese children the separation may be even greater, but by the age of 12 the legs should be straight. Separation of over 10 cm or unilateral knock knee requires an X-ray and, probably, a specialist opinion.

Scoliosis

A lateral curve of the spine is commonly seen in babies, and may be associated with skull asymmetry (plagiocephaly). Generally it is a postural scoliosis which goes when the baby is suspended and which has completely gone by the age of 2. Postural scoliosis is seen again at adolescence when it is commoner in girls; when the girl is asked to bend forward the curve straightens out. Fixed scoliosis at any age is likely to mean a vertebral or neurological abnormality.

Talipes (club foot)

Minor degrees of talipes are common at birth, resulting

Fig. 41. 'Physiological' bow legs in a 1-year-old. Two years later his legs looked straight.

from mechanical pressure in utero. The commonest deviation is that in which there is plantar flexion (equinus) and foot adduction (varus) at the midtarsal joint (Fig. 42). If the foot with talipes equino-varus can be fully dorsiflexed and everted so that the little toe touches the outside of the leg without undue force, it can be expected to correct itself with time. If it cannot be so overcorrected urgent splintage or surgery is needed. The sooner treatment is begun the better the outcome. Talipes

Talipes calcaneo-valgus   Talipes equino-varus

Fig. 42. Talipes

calcaneo-valgus describes the dorsiflexed foot which is everted so that the foot lies against the outer border of the leg with the little toe almost touching it. Usually the position is easily corrected by simple exercises.

Congenital defects of the spinal cord such as spina bifida cystica are commonly associated with severe talipes.

Congenital dislocation of the hip

Dislocated hips are associated with joint laxity and acetabular dysplasia. Postural factors play a role in their causation. They are commoner in:

—girls;
—babies presenting by the breech;
—full-term rather than pre-term babies;
—the left hip.

Diagnosis is made by specifically testing the hips: a modification of Ortolani's manoeuvre is one such test (Fig. 43). The baby is laid on its back with the feet towards the examiner. The legs are straightened. Then the examiner grasps the child's legs placing the middle finger of each hand on the outer aspects of each hip, and the thumb on the inner side. In turn each hip is half abducted and the leg is lifted up with the middle finger. A dislocated hip slips into the socket with a click. The dislocated hip does not abduct as fully as the normal hip. X-ray examination is unreliable in the first month. All babies should be

Fig. 43. Testing for dislocation of hips.

examined in the neonatal period and again at child health clinics during the first year.

One in 60 babies is found to have hip instability at birth; 85% recover spontaneously, but the remainder persist. Early splinting is successful within 2 months in most neonates. If undetected in the neonatal period it may not become apparent until the parents worry about their 2-year-old's limp. At that age treatment is more traumatic and less successful.

Osteogenesis imperfecta

This is a rare condition characterized by fragile bones and lax ligaments. In severe cases multiple fractures occur in utero, whilst milder cases may merely incur a few fractures between the ages of 4 and 14. Familial inheritance is common; affected children may have blue sclerotics and suffer deafness in adult life.

OSTEOMYELITIS (osteitis)

Pyogenic infection of bone is commoner in children than adults, and in boys than girls.

The usual site is the metaphysis of one of the long bones particularly in the legs. At all ages except infancy *Staphylococcus pyogenes* is by far the commonest pathogen. The sources of infection and portal of entry are uncertain.

It may present acutely with a high fever and localized pain. An infant may merely refuse to use the affected arm or leg. The cardinal sign of osteomyelitis is a localised point of acute bone tenderness. Over this there may be redness or oedema. There is a neutrophil leucocytosis. Blood culture usually identifies the organism responsible. X-ray is normal at first; it is only after 2 or more weeks that the signs of rarefaction and periosteal new bone formation may be seen. Osteomyelitis is a most serious condition in which the future growth of the bone is in jeopardy. Intensive treatment in hospital is needed. Large doses of antibiotics are given, and it is best to use an antibiotic which is effective against penicillin-resistant staphylococci, e.g. lincomycin or fusidic acid.

If treatment is given early, complete resolution occurs in most cases. If diagnosis is delayed surgical drainage is more likely to be needed.

Chronic osteomyelitis may result from inadequate treatment of acute osteomyelitis or trauma. There is persistent dull bone pain. X-ray shows necrotic areas of bone; it is these areas which harbour the bacteria. Radical surgery to remove necrotic tissue is combined with systemic antibiotics.

ARTHRITIS

Arthritis is characterized by a painful inflamed joint in which there is limitation of movement in all directions. Swelling is not always present. The joint itself is usually painful but occasionally the pain is referred to another area; hip pain may be referred to the knee.

The more important causes are:
1   Those which may result in permanent joint damage:
    (a) Juvenile rheumatoid arthritis (p. 196).
    (b) Acute suppurative arthritis due to blood-borne infection. This is treated with aspiration, antibiotics and splintage.
    (c) Tuberculosis and brucellosis, now very rare in developed countries.
2   Those which resolve completely (synovitis):
    (a) Trauma, especially in schoolchildren. In a child with hip pain and limp ('observation hip') only time may distinguish between trauma and Perthes' disease (see below).
    (b) Henoch–Schönlein syndrome (p. 197).

(c) Rheumatic fever (p. 195).
(d) Serum sickness and generalised allergic reactions.
(e) Viral infections, e.g.: rubella (and rubella immunization), mumps and chicken pox.

Haemarthrosis (bleeding into joints) in children with
coagulation disorders may mimic acute arthritis.

OSTEOCHONDRITIS AND EPIPHYSITIS

These terms are applied to bone changes which occur,
particularly in epiphyses of children, as a result of
avascular necrosis or excessive strain on a growing bone.
They present as bone pain, with local swelling and
tenderness. There is limitation of movement and adjacent
muscle wasting. Those that occur in weight bearing joints
are the most important, as permanent damage may occur.
The best example is *Perthes' disease* which affects the
femoral head of children (usually boys) aged 5–8 years. It
causes hip pain.

If the affected bone is not a weight-bearing one, the
consequences are minimal. Children aged 10–15 are
particularly prone to develop transient inflammation of
the tuberosity of the tibia and the patella. These resolve
satisfactorily with symptomatic treatment.

Further reading

Sharrard W. J. *Paediatric Orthopaedics and Fractures.* Blackwell
    Scientific Publications.
McKusick V. A. *Heritable Disorders of Connective Tissue.* C. V.
    Mosby.

Chapter 14

The Collagen Diseases

Rheumatic fever is primarily a condition of childhood. Rheumatoid arthritis, systemic lupus erythematosus and polyarteritis nodosa are primarily diseases of adults. Henoch–Schönlein syndrome is an important childhood condition and is grouped with the collagen diseases because of some similarities to them.

RHEUMATIC FEVER (acute rheumatism)

Rheumatic fever is still the most important cause of acquired heart disease in children throughout the world, but in Britain it has become rare and less severe. It is commoner in poor socioeconomic circumstances and occurs mainly between the ages of 5 to 15 years. There is a slight familial tendency. It results from a cross-sensitivity reaction to a β-haemolytic group A streptococcal infection. Typically there has been acute tonsillitis 1–6 weeks previously.

The child is ill and feverish. There may be severe abdominal or chest pain, and nose bleeds are common. The classical pathognomonic features are:

1 Polyarthritis. Medium-sized joints are affected—the knees, elbows and ankles. Pain 'flits' from joint to joint as the arthritis affects one joint for a day or two, and then affects another joint.

2 Carditis. Tachycardia and a short systolic murmur are usual. More certain evidence of cardiac involvement is a pansystolic or diastolic murmur, a pericardial friction rub or cardiac enlargement leading to cardiac failure.

3 Rashes. Erythema marginatum, a serpiginous red rash with a raised edge found most often on the trunk, is the

pathognomonic rash. Other rashes including erythema nodosum are commoner but not specific.

4   Nodules. Subcutaneous nodules, no bigger than a pea may be found over bony prominences. They are not tender.

5   Chorea. These involuntary movements are uncommon but may occur in older children up to 6 months after the original streptococcal infection.

Investigation of the blood shows a raised white cell count, and very high ESR and C reactive protein levels. Serial antistreptolysin O (ASO) titres show a sustained rise. The ECG may show conduction defects.

It is customary to impose bed-rest, particularly if there is heart involvement. Large doses of salicylates are the mainstay of drug treatment though corticosteroids may be used if there is carditis. A short course of penicillin is given followed by prolonged prophylaxis. Anyone who has had rheumatic fever is advised to take daily oral penicillin for life in order to reduce the chance of recurrence: 60% of patients are likely to develop rheumatic heart disease in later life, mitral stenosis being the outstanding complication.

JUVENILE CHRONIC ARTHRITIS

Under the age of 7 it presents in a characteristic way that may be called 'Still's disease'. Systemic features predominate; there is fever, splenomegaly, lymphadenopathy and transient rashes. Joint involvement may be comparatively mild. Although there is a raised ESR and white cell count, serum latex and Rose–Waaler tests are usually negative.

Over the age of 7 the adult pattern of illness (rheumatoid arthritis) is seen with joint involvement and little or no systemic upset. The main feature is the symmetrical involvement of both medium-sized joints and the small joints of the fingers, neck and temporo-mandibular joint (temporo-mandibular arthritis is pathognomonic of rheumatoid arthritis). However, in the early stages of the illness it may be difficult to differentiate from rheumatic fever.

At least 50% of children make a complete recovery, but the rest run a chronic relapsing course. Salicylates and physiotherapy are the mainstay of treatment, though more powerful drugs including indomethacin, gold and penicillamine may be required.

It is worth tissue typing children with chronic arthritis, particularly if the spine is involved, because the presence of HLA type B27 would suggest early onset of ankylosing spondylitis.

Other collagen diseases

Systemic lupus erythematosus (SLE), polyarteritis nodosa, dermatomyositis and the other collagen disorders are very rare in children. SLE is the least rare tending to occur in adolescent girls, particularly negroes. It tends to present as a multisystem disorder; many of the manifestations subside during treatment with corticosteroids, though neurological involvement may be particularly persistent.

HENOCH—SCHÖNLEIN SYNDROME
(anaphylactoid purpura, allergic purpura)

The syndrome is commonest in children aged 2–10 and is made up of a pathognomonic purpuric rash and involvement of one or more of the following: joints, alimentary system and kidneys.

Skin

The rash is distributed over extensor surfaces of the limbs, particularly about the ankles and on the buttocks (Fig. 44). It begins as a maculo-papular red rash, or as an urticarial rash in children under the age of 5, which gradually becomes purpuric. (The platelet count is normal.) Swelling of the face, hands and feet is common and subcutaneous bleeds may occur in the scrotum, eyelids and conjunctiva.

Joints

Pain (arthralgia) of medium-sized joints is common and may progress to an obvious arthritis with red, swollen, tender joints.

Fig. 44. Henoch–Schönlein purpura. The rash is symmetrically distributed and is most marked on the ankles, buttocks and extensor surfaces.

Alimentary system

Colicky abdominal pain occurs and may be severe enough to mimic an acute abdominal emergency. Vomiting and diarrhoea are common, haematemesis and melaena less common, and intussusception or perforation very rare.

Kidneys

Microscopic haematuria and transient proteinuria are common. With more severe involvement the glomerulo-nephritis causes an acute nephritic syndrome, a nephrotic syndrome or renal insufficiency. The renal complications are responsible for the main morbidity and mortality of Henoch–Schönlein syndrome.

The various groups of symptoms generally present within a week of each other, but may occur in any order and persist for several weeks. Recurrence of any symptoms may occur for several months after onset. The cause is unknown and treatment is symptomatic.

Further reading

Hughes G. V. R. *Connective Tissue Diseases*, Blackwell Scientific Publications.

Chapter 15

The Skin

Skin disorders are a common reason for children being taken to the doctor. The infant's skin with its thin epidermis and immature glands is particularly liable to infection and blistering. Birthmarks, napkin rashes, infections and eczema are common in pre-school children. Thereafter the incidence of skin disease declines until adolescence when acne is common.

BIRTHMARKS

Birthmarks may be the result of (a) developmental anomalies of the blood vessels—naevi or haemangiomas, or (b) an excess of pigment in the skin.

(a) The main types of naevi are:

Stork mark (naevus flammeus) (Fig. 45)

This is a flat pinkish capillary haemangioma at the nape of the neck and also between the eyebrows of the infant (as if the stork had pecked the baby with its beak). It appears more red when the baby cries, but fades gradually during the first 2 years.

Strawberry naevus (Fig. 46)

This is a soft raised bright red capillary haemangioma often containing or overlying a more bluish cavernous haemangioma. It is not apparent until a few days after birth, and usually enlarges during the first 6 months. Thereafter sunken whitish areas develop in the lump and it gradually becomes paler and flatter. Most have disappeared by the age of 7 years, so that surgery or other

Fig. 45 Stork mark. This capillary haemangioma characteristically lies just above the nose. The upper eyelids are quite commonly affected as in this baby.

treatment is best reserved for the very few which are extremely unsightly, do not regress spontaneously, or are expanding rapidly. In general spontaneous regression does not leave a noticeable scar, whilst treatment often does (Fig. 47).

Port wine stain

Port wine stain is a capillary haemangioma which forms a flat dark purple patch of skin which looks ugly. It does not fade. Treatment is difficult, and camouflage with cosmetics is often the best treatment. *Sturge–Weber syndrome* is a rare association of a unilateral port wine stain of the face (including the areas supplied by the first division of the trigeminal nerve) and an intracranial haemangioma of the pia-arachnoid on the same side. Affected children may present with fits or neurological signs (p. 89).

Fig. 46. A strawberry naevus.

(b) Small **pigmented birthmarks** (pigmented moles) usually develop after the age of 2. They are common and rarely cause anxiety to parents.

Mongolian blue spots

These are large blue-grey areas most common over the sacrum and buttocks, which look rather like bruises (Fig. 48). They are only found in infants of Oriental, Asian or Negro stock, and gradually fade so that they are rarely visible after the age of 5.

Fig. 47. A massive capillary haemangioma. The paler areas represent the start of spontaneous resolution.

RASHES

Napkin rash

Eruptions of the napkin area are common in infants. Characteristically an erythematous rash affects the convexities of the buttocks, inner thighs and genitalia. The skin creases, which do not come into contact with the nappy, are spared (Fig. 49). At its simplest it may merely

Fig. 48. A Mongolian blue spot over the sacrum. A smaller darker spot is present over the right iliac crest.

be an irritant rash caused by abrasive napkins or wetness. Fresh urine does not injure the skin, but prolonged contact with stale urine which has broken down to form ammonia products does (ammoniacal dermatitis). In severe cases (Fig. 50) papules and vesicles form which ulcerate, leaving a moist surface which easily becomes secondarily infected with either pyogenic organisms or monilia. Secondary infection with monilia usually does involve the skin creases. It causes a moist erythematous rash with oval macules and vesicles, a pimply margin and scattered sattelite papules.

It is impossible for mothers to change their baby's nappy immediately it is wet. Nappy rashes occur in all classes of society and are not simply confined to babies who have poor care. Some babies have a more sensitive skin than others, and are prone to develop the rash. This must be explained to the mother to dispel needless guilt. However, gross ulcerated and chronic napkin rashes are a sign of inadequate care.

The skin may be irritated by specific detergents and

Fig. 49. Napkin rash—most prominent on the convexities. The involvement of skin creases and the pimply margin suggest secondary monilial infection.

softening solutions used by the mother. Careful questioning is needed to eliminate the possibility of such a chemical rash.

Treatment is based on the mother carrying out as many of the following instructions as are practicable: frequent and prompt changing of wet nappies including washing and drying the baby's perineum carefully; thorough washing of the nappies using a final rinse in an antiseptic such as cetrimide; rubbing a barrier cream or benzalkonium cream on the napkin area; avoiding plastic pants until the rash is cured as these create a hot steamy environment inside; using a 'nappy liner'—a thin specially treated piece of material which transmits moisture to the nappy but remains dry itself. In severe cases the most effective treatment is exposure of the moist rash in a warm dry environment, leaving the nappies off for a few days, together with the use of hydrocortisone cream to

Fig. 50. Severe napkin rash with secondary ulceration.

suppress the inflammation. Secondary infection requires local bactericidal or fungicidal cream.

The possibility of *seborrhoeic dermatitis* should be considered in any young infant presenting with a napkin eruption who also has a rash of the groins, axilla and neck. The post-auricular region may be involved, but not the cheeks. Steroid treatment is helpful; secondary infection is common. The rash, which is usually not itchy, disappears by the age of 8 months.

Cradle cap

Cradle cap is as common in infants as dandruff and scurf are in older children. It is a thick, light brown crust over the top of the scalp which may look quite difficult to remove. Most chemists sell proprietary brands of medicated shampoo ('cradle cap remover') with which to wash the baby's scalp; alternatively salicylic acid and sulphur cream may be rubbed in before washing the hair. Regular washing of the scalp helps to prevent recurrence.

Eczema

This is common in atopic children whose families give a history of asthma, eczema or hay fever. The skin of atopic children is short of protolipids and this predisposes to eczema; the child is also at risk for asthma and hay fever. The erythematous scaling rash usually appears before the age of 6 months, and in infants generally involves the face, scalp and trunk (infantile eczema—Fig. 51).

(a)   (b)

Fig. 51. Distribution of eczema.
(a) infancy: cheeks, scalp and behind ears are commonly affected.
(b) later childhood: skin flexures, particularly antecubital and popliteal fossae.

There is intense itching, and scratching frequently leads to secondary infection (Fig. 52). The condition fluctuates, resolves completely in half the children by the age of 2, but in others persists in a mild form or periodically recurs. After infancy the rash is characteristically distributed in the skin flexures, particularly in the antecubital and popliteal fossae (flexural eczema—Fig. 51).

Fig. 52. Infantile eczema involving the face and leading to secondary bacterial infection.

Prolonged inflammation leads to thick lichenified skin and local lymph gland enlargement.

Frequent bathing in a bath to which emulsifying oil or ointment has been added is followed by the local application of steroid ointment or tar paste. Bactericidal creams are used for secondary infection. Antihistamines, particularly trimeprazine, subdue the itching. Other measures may include hypnotics at night, and restraining clothing such as cloth mittens which are then fastened to the cot side to prevent the infant scratching. The condition tends to improve, and certainly becomes more manageable as the child becomes older.

Psoriasis

This unpleasant skin condition is commonest at the age of 10–11 and in the early 40s. Autosomal dominant inheritance is usual, and at all ages stress seems to be a provocative factor. The typical lesions are silvery scales on top of a circumscribed salmon red base. Most types affect principally the extensor surface of the limbs and the scalp; they do not itch. The guttate variety, found mainly on the trunk, appears 2–3 weeks after a streptococcal infection such as tonsillitis. Coal tar ointment and shampoo is the treatment of choice.

Impetigo

This is a skin infection which may start with a streptococcus, but by the time it reaches the doctor is usually staphylococcal. It commonly involves the face, around the mouth and nose, and the hands. It begins as a small red spot which rapidly ulcerates, producing exudate which dries in a golden brown crust over the red itching skin beneath. Spread may be rapid and scratching may spread it to other parts of the body or to other members of the family. It is very contagious, so the child should be excluded from school until it is healed. Impetigo frequently complicates herpes simplex or infestation with scabies or pediculosis.

The lesions respond fast to bathing with cetrimide and water to remove the crusts, and a short course of oral erythromycin. The family must be warned about the risk of becoming infected themselves and the affected child should use a separate towel and face cloth.

Warts

Warts are most common in childhood, probably because of the opportunity for contact spread of the responsible virus. The average life of a wart is 3–4 months, so treatment is usually reserved for long-lasting warts. The variety of available treatments and magic cures are a fair indication of the therapeutic problem and the variable natural history. Children with a plantar wart (*verruca*) are sometimes banned from swimming baths. However, the prevalence of verrucas and the chance of their transmission are so high that banning the occasional affected child is unlikely to be helpful.

Urticaria (hives)

Urticaria is common in children, especially under the age of 5. It is characterized by red blotches and whitish wheals which itch. They disappear and reappear over a period of hours or days. Sometimes sensitivity to a particular drug or food appears to be responsible. Treatment is symptomatic; systemic antihistamines or adrenaline may produce dramatic relief. *Papular urticaria* consists of hard papules most often on the limbs. They appear in crops and itch so that secondary infection is common. In many children they are associated with insect bites, fleas, lice and bed bugs. In Britain papular urticaria is particularly common in the late summer.

Erythema nodosum

The shiny red lumps are 1–3 cm in diameter and may be extremely tender. They are most commonly distributed symmetrically over the front of the shins, but do occur elsewhere. During the first week they become more protuberant, purple and painful, then during the next 2 weeks gradually subside and look like old bruises. They may occur at intervals in crops. Although they are thought to represent a hypersensitivity phenomenon to certain stimuli, the provocative stimulus frequently cannot be identified. In childhood the important associations are:
1   Streptococcal infection;
2   Tuberculosis;
3   Certain drugs;
4   Rare childhood diseases such as sarcoidosis, lupus erythematosus and ulcerative colitis.

INFESTATIONS

Pediculosis

The commonest louse infestation in childhood is with the

head louse (*pediculosis capitis*). The louse lives in the hair and lives off blood which it gets by biting the scalp. It causes irritation, and the combination of the bites and the child scratching frequently leads to impetigo and enlarged occipital and cervical lymph glands. The bites may resemble purpura confined to the neck and shoulders. Sometimes the lice can be seen, but more often just the tiny whitish eggs (nits) are seen attached singly to the hair. They can be identified with certainty beneath a microscope; they are ovoid with one blunt end and one pointed end by which they are stuck to the hair shaft. Applications of malathion or carbaryl lotion are rubbed into the hair and left overnight before it is washed. Other members of the home should be examined for similar infestations.

Scabies

The mite *Sarcoptes scabiei* lays its eggs in burrows beneath the skin. The larva migrates and burrows into the skin, gradually developing into the adult mite, which re-emerges, becomes impregnated and burrows to lay more eggs. After a few weeks the child becomes sensitized and develops a very itchy papulovesicular rash. In older children this is most marked in the interdigital spaces, wrist flexures and anterior axillary folds. In infants it frequently involves the face, trunk and feet. The burrows can be seen as small linear elevations of skin adjacent to a small vesicle, but they are often obscured by excoriation and secondary infection. Diagnosis is confirmed by microscopic identification of a mite from one of the burrows. Scabies has become increasingly common in Britain and should be considered as a possible cause for any unexplained itching rash. The infestation is transferred by bodily contact, so that other members of the family are usually affected, and all those living together should be treated at the same time. One or two applications of gamma benzene hexachloride are required and disinfestation of clothing and bedding is advised.

Chapter 16

The Urinary Tract

DEVELOPMENT

The fetus excretes urine from the 12th week of intrauterine life, and by term it is both swallowing and excreting 500 ml/day. This function is more important for the production of amniotic fluid than for elimination of waste products, since the fetus is being effectively haemodialysed by the placenta.

At birth renal function is limited. The baby can cope well with normal food intake simply because body growth is rapid and milk contains exactly the right substances required for growth with little excess. When this situation is altered the limitations of the immature kidney are seen. If the neonate has excess intravenous fluid it becomes oedematous. If it has diarrhoea the kidneys fail to conserve fluid adequately. Compared with the adult a relatively small decrease in renal perfusion, e.g. from mild dehydration or cardiac failure, may result in a raised plasma urea level.

Although glomerular function is limited during the first year it is more efficient than tubular function. Morphologically the glomeruli, which are half adult size at birth, are relatively larger than the tubules. As the kidney matures tubular growth and function increase faster so that by the age of 1 year the adult balance is present. Renal growth continues throughout childhood by means of increase in nephron size, and not by the production of new nephrons. A steady increase of size of renal outline, as seen on X-ray, is a useful sign of healthy growing kidneys.

The child's kidney is relatively larger than the adult and on X-ray the length should be equivalent to the length of four mid-lumbar vertebrae plus discs.

URINE EXAMINATION

Routine examination includes inspection, smell, chemical test and microscopy. Careful collection of a fresh specimen, preferably mid-stream, into a clean container is necessary.

1 *Inspection*

(a) Translucency. Fresh urine should appear clear when held up to the light. Chemical deposits are the commonest reason for a cloudy appearance (particularly in cold stale urine); phosphates disappear if 2 drops of dilute acetic acid are added; urates and other acid salts tend to dissolve on gentle warming. Infected urine is usually hazy, and can be frankly cloudy. If the urine is crystal clear it is unlikely to be infected.

(b) Colour. The main influence on colour is the concentration of the urine, dilute urine from someone who has drunk a lot being almost colourless. Blood may appear obviously red but more commonly appears pinkish or reddish-brown sometimes with a 'smoky' tint. Ingested foods, confectionery and drugs are common reasons for unusual colours.

(c) Frothiness. When the container is shaken gently normal urine settles fast without much froth. Frothiness is a feature of protein or bile in the urine.

2 *Smell*

In some urine infections urea-splitting organisms produce a foul fishy smell. This is also the smell of stale urine which has been left standing in a warm place. Some foods and drugs produce characteristic odours (e.g. penicillin). Chemicals produced by body metabolism also influence urine smell: ketones commonly, and products of inborn errors of metabolism very rarely—because those diseases are extremely rare. (For connoisseurs of smells there is one syndrome that produces a 'sweaty feet' urine, and another that produces 'maple syrup' urine.)

3 *Chemical tests*

The most convenient are the chemically impregnated

paper or plastic test strips ('dipstix'). These should be used according to the directions on the packet. The stix is immersed momentarily in the urine, the surplus urine is dislodged by tapping it and the colour change of the indicator paper is noted at the stipulated time. That time interval is critical for some tests, e.g. haemoglobin. It is important to check that the stix is held the right way round to compare appropriately with the illustrative label on the container. Of the many dipstix tests available the more important for children are:

(a) *Albumin*: 20% of children have a trace of albumin in their urine, it can be disregarded; 5% have 0·3 g/l or more. If this is persistent a 24-hour collection is made; an excretion of over 0·3 g/day requires further investigation. Transient albuminuria may occur with fever or hard exercise.

(b) *Glucose*: likely causes are a low renal threshold or hyperglycaemia, e.g. diabetes mellitus. (*Clinistix* is specific for glucose. *Clinitest* is a modified Benedict test in tablet form, and detects any reducing sugar.) In the first 2 weeks of life small amounts of glucose and other reducing sugars are commonly found in the urine.

(c) *Haemoglobin*: even though the test is extremely sensitive and may be positive when there is no tint of blood visible on looking at the urine, positive reactions are always abnormal. The usual cause is haematuria. Since haemoglobinuria and myoglobinuria produce a positive test also, microscopy is mandatory.

(d) *pH*: the usual pH is 5 or 6. Alkaline urine is more likely in infants than in older children because of the frequent feeds; it also occurs after alkaline medicines and sometimes in the presence of urine infection.

(e) *Ketones*: this test is present on most dipstix, but it is of limited value since ketonuria is common in children who are ill, anorexic or have been vomiting, or in the many school children who have no breakfast.

4   *Microscopy*

Regardless of the precise method used, microscopic examination of urine is a most valuable skill. Some people use a counting chamber in order to record the number of formed elements per mm^3 of unspun urine. Others centrifuge the urine and enumerate it (less accurately) per high power field. There is no reliable standard for converting cells per high power field of centrifuged urine to cells per mm^3 of unspun urine. The urine should be examined under low power with fairly low illumination before increasing the illumination to examine under high power. Constant 'racking' of the fine focus is needed, since the specimen is deeper than a histological specimen.

White blood cells (WBC, pus cells). A healthy boy may have up to 5 WBC/mm^3 and a girl up to 50/mm^3 (unspun). Excess cells (pyuria) may be the result of a urine infection or an abnormality of the renal tract (Fig. 53).

Red blood cells (RBC). These may be difficult to identify because they lose their round shape fast and haemolyse. Urine should not contain more than 2 RBC/mm^3. The commonest causes of haematuria are glomerulonephritis and urinary tract infection. Casts should be searched for to localise the site of the blood loss.

Casts. These are formed in the renal tubules. Cellular casts may be composed of renal tubular cells, but more commonly are composed of red cells, or disintegrating red

Fig. 53. Gross pyuria. The urine contained more than 40,000 WBC/mm^3, many of them aggregated in clumps. The granular appearance of nucleated white cells is visible on either low- or high-power microscopy.

cells (granular casts). They are an important sign of glomerulonephritis. Hyaline casts devoid of cells are invariably present whenever there is proteinuria, and a few may be present in a concentrated early morning specimen from a normal child.

Bacteria. If the urine is infected bacteria can usually be seen as motile rods, even in unspun unstained urine using the low-power objective. They can be identified more certainly under high power (Fig. 54).

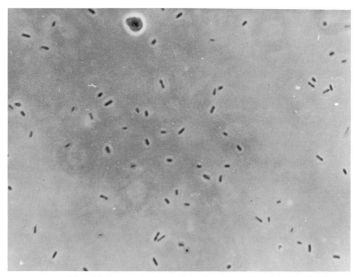

Fig. 54. Bacteriuria. Infected urine viewed under high power; many of the organisms were motile. There is a white cell at the top of the picture.

CONGENITAL ANOMALIES

Agenesis

This is the result of the ureteric bud failing to develop so that the ureter and kidney are absent. If unilateral the child may live a full and healthy life provided the other kidney is normal. Bilateral agenesis is lethal. Oligohydramnios has usually been noted during pregnancy, and a proportion of affected infants have a characteristic facial appearance (Potter's syndrome).

Hypoplastic kidneys

These are deficient in renal parenchyma. They are not usually associated with other abnormalities.

Dysplastic kidneys

These contain abnormally differentiated parenchyma. They are commonly associated with obstruction and other abnormalities of the urinary tract. *Polycystic disease* represents one form of renal dysplasia. Infantile polycystic disease is associated with massive kidneys, renal failure early in life and a recessive pattern of inheritance, whereas adult polycystic disease which has a dominant inheritance is generally not detected in early life because the kidneys are not enlarged and function well during childhood.

Ureteric abnormalities

Obstruction is commonest at the pelvi-ureteric junction where it may cause hydronephrosis and permanent renal damage. *Duplication* of the ureter and pelvis may occur on one or both sides. If it only affects the upper half of the ureter it is not important, but if it extends down to the bladder so that there are two separate ureteric openings on that side there are commonly abnormalities of the lower ureter. A *ureterocele* is a cystic enlargement of the ureter within the bladder which may cause obstruction.

Bladder and urethral abnormalities

Posterior urethral valves

These are an important cause of obstruction to urine flow and occur almost exclusively in boys. Bladder neck obstruction is more rare. They usually present in the newborn period or at least in the first year as acute obstruction or chronic partial obstruction with dribbling micturition.

N.B. Obstruction of the lower urinary tract is frequently associated with renal dysplasia. But regardless of potential renal function, obstruction may cause direct damage by back pressure or predispose to urinary tract infection which may cause further damage. Most obstructive abnormalities can be corrected by surgery.

Hypospadias

The urethral opening is on the ventral surface of the penis (Fig. 55). If it is at the junction of the glans and shaft no treatment is needed, but if it is on the shaft of the penis plastic surgery is required before school entry. The foreskin may be needed for this reconstruction, therefore boys with hypospadias should not be circumcised. In all but the mildest cases there is ventral flexion (*chordee*) of the penis. There may be associated meatal stenosis.

Fig. 55. Hypospadias. The meatus is at the junction of the glans and shaft. The prepuce is characteristically misshapen and hooded.

RENAL DISEASE

Terminology and classification

In recent years nephrologists have begun to use the same language as each other. This is a major advance, and the starting point for understanding renal disease is to appreciate the classifications that are used.

Firstly, syndromes—collections of symptoms and signs, are defined, e.g. nephrotic syndrome or acute nephritic syndrome.

Secondly, a pathological or morphological description is given. This is obtained from biopsy or autopsy, e.g. proliferative glomerulonephritis or 'minimal changes'.

Thirdly, an aetiological label is added when this is known, e.g. 'diabetic' or 'post-streptococcal'.

Whilst there are certain correlations between these three levels of diagnosis, it is essential to realise that a particular morphological appearance (for instance, proliferative glomerulonephritis) may be found in each of several different clinical syndromes. Further, a syndrome may be associated with several different morphological pictures, and have a variety of different aetiologies.

The most important syndromes of renal disease in childhood are:
Acute nephritic syndrome;
Recurrent haematuria;
Nephrotic syndrome;
Symptomless proteinuria;
Urinary tract infection;
Renal insufficiency.

ACUTE NEPHRITIC SYNDROME

This is characterized by haematuria, oliguria, hypertension and a raised plasma urea. The last two features are not always present.

Aetiology

The best-known form is post-streptococcal glomerulonephritis, sometimes called acute nephritis. The child has had a beta-haemolytic streptococcal infection, usually a pharyngitis, 2–3 weeks previously. Immune complexes composed of streptococci, antibody and complement are deposited in the glomeruli. There they provoke proliferation of the endothelial cells (proliferative glomerulonephritis). Post-streptococcal glomerulonephritis which was once a common condition is now uncommon in Britain.

An acute nephritic syndrome may also occur at the time of pneumococcal pneumonia, septicaemia and some viral infections. It is sometimes seen in Henoch–Schönlein syndrome and the collagen diseases.

Features

Acute nephritic syndrome has an age distribution with a peak at 7 years. The child is well until the sudden onset of illness and the appearance of bright red or brownish urine. Facial oedema, particularly of the eyelids, is common, and there may be abdominal or loin pain together with loin tenderness. The blood pressure is raised in half the children.

Investigations

A small volume of blood-stained urine is passed. In addition to copious red blood cells there is an excess of white cells and proteinuria. Red cell and granular casts are present.

The blood urea is raised in two-thirds of children. Serial antistreptolysin O (ASO) titres show a rise to above 1:250. Serum C_3 complement is reduced for 2–8 weeks after onset.

Course and treatment

Oliguria lasts for only a few days. Diuresis usually occurs within a week and is accompanied by return of plasma urea and blood pressure to normal. The haematuria and proteinuria gradually subside over the next year or so.

During the oliguric phase fluid and protein are restricted, but it is rarely necessary to start a strict renal failure regime. Penicillin is given for 3 months to reduce the chance of recurrence, which in any case is rare. Other treatment is symptomatic; the child is kept in bed only as long as he feels ill.

Over 80% make a full recovery, but a few develop progressive renal disease. Death in the acute phase from hypertensive encephalopathy, cardiac failure or acute renal failure is very rare.

RECURRENT HAEMATURIA SYNDROME

It is characterized by recurrent bouts of haematuria. These may occur at the time of a systemic infection or exertion. The child may feel mildly unwell but more often has no symptoms. The haematuria results from nephritis of unknown cause.

Between attacks the urine is normal or shows microscopic haematuria. Proteinuria is less common and may indicate more serious renal disease.

Investigations are done to exclude other causes of haematuria: urine culture, intravenous urogram (IVU/IVP) for a tumour or stone, and screening tests for bleeding disorders. If, as is usual, the urine contains red cell and granular casts cystoscopy constitutes an improper assault, since casts originate from the kidneys.

The prognosis is good. Renal function is normal and continues so in over 90%. The bouts of haematuria may continue for several years, and the doctor who has the task of reassuring the parents usually ends up wishing that blood was colourless. Prolonged restriction of activity or bed rest is more likely to result in an uneducated delinquent adolescent than to affect the renal prognosis.

NEPHROTIC SYNDROME

Nephrotic syndrome is characterized by heavy proteinuria, hypoalbuminaemia and oedema.

Features

It is commonest in boys aged 2–3 years. Apart from the gradual onset of generalized oedema the child may be well or only mildly off colour. Other symptoms are directly related to oedema, for instance discomfort from ascites or breathlessness from pleural effusion (Fig. 56).

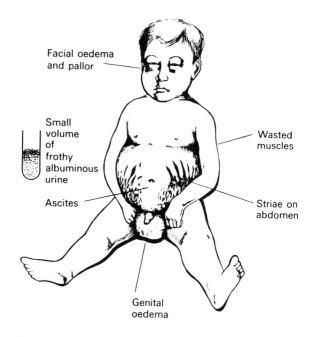

Fig. 56. Nephrotic syndrome.

Facial oedema and pallor

Small volume of frothy albuminous urine

Ascites

Wasted muscles

Striae on abdomen

Genital oedema

Aetiology

Over 90% of childhood nephrotic syndrome is the result of primary renal disease of unknown cause. Nephrotic syndrome secondary to systemic illness is less common than in adults, the least rare causes being Henoch–Schön-lein syndrome and the collagen diseases. In Africa, quartan malaria is an important cause.

Pathology

Up to the age of 5 years 80% of affected children will show only 'minimal changes'. This means that the biopsy appearance is nearly normal on light microscopy and that there is no significant immunofluorescent staining. After the age of 10 more serious pathology becomes likely.

Investigations

The urine is frothy and albuminous. The 24-hour excretion of protein is anything from 1 to 20 g. Highly selective proteinuria, that is urine containing a high proportion of small molecular weight proteins, is a good prognostic feature suggesting minimal change histology. Hyaline casts are abundant. Serum albumin is below 25 g/l and the serum cholesterol is usually raised. Plasma urea is normal.

Treatment and prognosis

A high protein, low salt diet is given, and moderate fluid restriction imposed. Corticosteroids are given in large doses for 4–6 weeks. Diuretics may be needed if the oedema is causing symptoms. Most children go into remission within 2 weeks of starting steroids. Diuresis occurs and the oedema and albuminuria disappear rapidly. A large proportion relapse within the next year. They can be given further courses of steroids, but if the relapses are frequent cyclophosphamide will usually produce a longer remission.

The long-term prognosis is better than it is for adults with nephrotic syndrome. Most children are well and have normal renal function 10 years later. A small proportion, including many of those initially unresponsive to steroids, develop renal insufficiency. Unusual

Table 12. Comparison of findings in acute nephritic syndrome, nephrotic syndrome and urinary tract infection

		Acute nephritic syndrome	Nephrotic syndrome	Urinary tract infection
Child	Oedema	Mild facial	Gross	None
	Blood pressure	Raised	Normal	Normal
Urine	Albumen	+ +	+ + + +	+ or 0
	RBC	+ + + +	0	+ or 0
	WBC	+ +	0	+ / + + +
	Casts	Cellular/granular	Hyaline	0
	Bacteria	0	0	+ + + +

223

features at onset which are unfavourable prognostic signs are: late age of onset, haematuria, hypertension or raised plasma urea. Renal biopsy tends to be reserved for children showing these features.

SYMPTOMLESS PROTEINURIA

Persistent proteinuria with a urinary excretion of more than 0·3 g/day is abnormal (see p. 214). It may be a sign of renal disease, and requires investigation. Before embarking on elaborate tests of renal function or a biopsy it is important to exclude postural (orthostatic) proteinuria, since this is commonest in the age range 10–15 years. Such children do not have proteinuria when recumbent in bed, but have excess proteinuria when up and active, particularly after adopting an excessively lordotic position. Postural proteinuria is generally considered a benign condition which does not progress.

URINARY TRACT INFECTION

Infection of the urinary tract is one of the commonest and most puzzling conditions of childhood. Because it is unusual to be able to localize the infection to any particular site it is preferable to call it 'urinary tract infection' than to use words such as 'cystitis' or 'pyelitis'.

Incidence

From birth to adolescence the prevalence of urinary tract infection is just over 1%. In the neonatal period boys are more often infected, but thereafter girls predominate. By the age of 2 years, 5% of girls have had a urinary tract infection, and during the school years infection is 25 times more likely in a girl.

Pathology

The commonest pathogen is *E. coli*. Bacteria of the same strain are usually present in the child's gut and it is assumed that the organism enters the urethra via the perineum.

Features

The child may have neither symptoms nor signs. When there are symptoms they tend to be non-specific: feeding problems, fever, prolonged jaundice in the neonate; vague malaise, enuresis or urgency in the older child. The classical adult picture of burning dysuria, fever and loin pain is uncommon in children.

Investigations

The diagnosis is made if a carefully collected clean specimen of urine contains more than 10^8 organisms/l in pure growth. A mixed growth is more likely to be the result of contamination than infection. A colony count of less than 10^7/l is normal, a count in between means that the culture must be repeated. Ideally a positive diagnosis should not be made unless two consecutive colony counts have contained more than 10^8 organisms/l. The greatest problem in infants is obtaining a clean urine sample. Self-adhesive perineal plastic bags are widely used; they must be emptied immediately urine has been passed to avoid perineal contamination. Children's wards sometimes use wet (or warm)-sensitive electronic devices for notifying the nurses as soon as micturition occurs. Such 'squirt-alerts' or 'pee-peepers' allow fresh urine to be collected and despatched promptly for culture. Occasionally it is necessary to resort to supra-pubic aspiration of urine directly from the bladder using a syringe and needle. The infant's bladder lies relatively high above the pubis so that it is not difficult to aspirate.

Macroscopically the urine may have an opalescent sheen. Microscopically bacteria are seen (usually motile rods) and there may be an excess of white cells. The presence of albuminuria is irrelevant to diagnosis. Haematuria may be present.

Management

1 Initial treatment. Fluid intake is increased and frequent micturition encouraged. Appropriate chemotherapy is given for 5 days; sulphonamides are effective, safe and inexpensive.

2   Further investigation. Ideally an intravenous urogram should be done on any child who has had a definite
urinary infection. The aim is to detect obstructive abnormalities. This is followed by a micturating cystogram in
many cases. Vesicoureteric reflux is found in a quarter of
cases: as the bladder empties, urine refluxes up the ureter
and at the end of micturition falls back to form a stagnant
residual pool (Fig. 57). Older children may be advised to

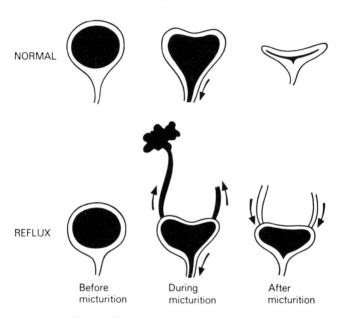

NORMAL

REFLUX

Before   During   After
micturition   micturition   micturition

Fig. 57. Vesico-ureteric reflux. At the end of micturition there
remains in the bladder a puddle of stagnant urine.

practice 'double micturition', trying to void the residual
pool a minute or so after each act of micturition. It is a
difficult trick, and it may be more realistic merely to
advise increased fluid intake and increased frequency of
micturition. Reflux is commoner in children than in
adults, and providing recurrent infections can be prevented, for instance by prophylactic antibiotics, it tends
to go as the child grows. If medical treatment is unsuc-
226   cessful, surgical correction of the reflux is possible.

3 Follow-up is the most important part of the management. One-third of children will have a recurrence within the next year. It is as unrealistic to claim having 'cured' a urine infection on the basis of sterile urine 2 days after treatment as it would be to claim having 'cured' an asthmatic child on the basis of having stopped one bout of wheezing. The child's urine must be cultured a few days after completing the initial 7 days' therapy, and 1, 3, 6 and 12 months afterwards, *even though the child is symptomless.*

The problem of prognosis

Infection of the renal parenchyma may cause permanent or progressive damage leading to renal insufficiency. Although radiologists sometimes describe such small scarred kidneys as 'chronic pyelonephritis' a truer morphological label is chronic interstitial nephritis. The same morphological appearance is seen in the later stages of renal disease of many origins other than infection. It is clear that the vast majority of the multitude of children with urinary tract infection do not incur renal damage. Renal damage is most likely in those with recurrent infection and ureteric reflux under the age of 5. But this is a large group of girls and most of them, even though they may have infections throughout childhood, have a fate no worse than 'honeymoon cystitis' and acute pyelonephritis of pregnancy.

We have no way of identifying the tiny minority whose kidneys are destined to be damaged by infection. Therefore, as bacterial infection may be one of the few preventable causes of chronic renal insufficiency an active policy has to be followed to detect, treat and follow-up children with urinary tract infections.

RENAL CALCULI

Stones in the urinary tract of children are less common than in adults. Occasionally they cause pain or renal colic but more often are detected by chance on X-ray. Most stones are of infective origin, especially in boys with a proteus infection. Since they can be of metabolic origin it is customary to check the urine for abnormal amino-acids (e.g. cystinuria) and the serum calcium and phosphate.

RENAL INSUFFICIENCY (RENAL FAILURE)

Acute renal failure describes the situation in which previously healthy kidneys suddenly stop working. It is a rewarding condition to treat in childhood because a higher proportion of children have recoverable conditions than do adults who present acutely.

A particularly notorious form is the haemolytic–uraemic syndrome which affects mainly older infants and toddlers. After a brief gastroenteritis-like illness the child presents with a haemolytic anaemia, thrombocytopenia and acute renal failure. Early peritoneal dialysis and expert management in a paediatric renal unit enable more than 80% to survive and recover good renal function.

Progressive renal insufficiency or chronic renal failure is uncommon in children. During the early months of life congenital abnormalities, particularly renal dysplasia, are the main cause. Thereafter primary renal diseases (various forms of glomerulonephritis) are the commonest cause. Children with end-stage renal disease have the same features as adults, e.g. anaemia, hypertension and renal rickets; in addition they fail to grow. Facilities for regular dialysis and transplantation for children are available in most regions of Britain. At present a selective policy is being used, long-term maintenance therapy only being offered to children who have reached school age.

Further reading

James J. A. *Renal Disease in Childhood*. C. V. Mosby.
Williams D. I. *Paediatric Urology*. Butterworths.
Edelmann C. M. *Paediatric Kidney Disease*. Little, Brown.

Chapter 17

The Blood

The normal blood picture

The neonate has a haemoglobin of 19 g/dl (130%). Erythropoiesis is limited during the early months, so that the haemoglobin level falls (Table 13). It reaches its lowest level of 11 g/dl (75%) at 3 months and thereafter rises steadily. These levels are normal at that age and therefore it is better to express children's haemoglobin levels as 'x g/dl' rather than as a percentage of the normal adult level. Red cell size (MCV) is large at birth, low at 1 year and rises to the adult level at puberty; a low MCV is a useful sign of iron deficiency or of thalassaemia trait. At birth haemoglobin is mainly of the fetal type—HbF. This combines more readily with oxygen at low oxygen tensions, and also gives up CO_2 more easily than does HbA, the adult type. During the first year HbF is gradually replaced by HbA. The white cell count is relatively higher throughout childhood, and in the early years there is a preponderance of lymphocytes which is particularly marked during the first year. Leucocytosis in response to infection is also more marked, and occasionally includes a few primitive white cells. In infants a lymphocytic response to infection does not exclude a bacterial cause. The platelet count is mildly reduced in the first few months but by 6 months the normal adult value of $250–350 \times 10^9/l$ is reached. The ESR should be below 16 in childhood, provided that the packed cell volume is at least 35%.

ANAEMIA

Anaemia is common in childhood, but not quite as common as many mothers suspect. Mothers are often

Table 13. Normal blood picture

Age	Haemoglobin (g/dl)	Type	MCV	WBC ($\times 10^9$/l)	Lymphocytes (%)
1–2 weeks	18	HbF > HbA	96	12·0	70
1 month	15	HbF > HbA	91	11·0	65
3 months	12	HbF < HbA	84	11·0	65
1 year	12	HbA	78	10·0	55
4 years	13	HbA	80	9·0	40
12 years	14	HbA	81	8·0	30

worried by their child's pallor, which is more often a feature of a fair complexion than of anaemia. Anaemia may cause tiredness and even breathlessness, but most tired children are not anaemic. Examination of the mucous membranes is more reliable than skin colour, but whenever anaemia is suspected a blood test is necessary. It is imperative to report back to parents that a blood test is normal; many parents think a blood test is being done because the doctor suspects leukaemia.

Anaemia may be caused by:
1 Diminished production
2 Excessive breakdown
3 Blood loss.

1 Diminished production

(a) Deficiency anaemias

Iron deficiency anaemia is by far the most common, and is characterised by a hypochromic microcytic blood picture (Fig. 58). Reduction in MCV is a useful early sign, and is followed by a reduction of mean corpuscular haemoglobin concentration to less than 32 g/dl. Basically it is caused by insufficient intake of iron, which is more common in the following groups of children:
  (i) Pre-term babies and twins (p. 32).
 (ii) Infants who have to exist entirely on milk and are late changing to iron-containing weaning foods—sometimes because the infant is retarded or has cerebral palsy and is late learning to chew solids.

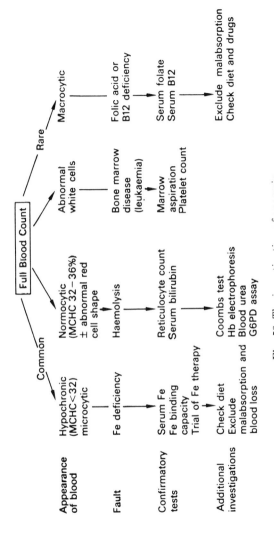

Fig. 58. The investigation of anaemia.

(iii) Children from homes where poverty, ignorance, or religious/racial factors prevent the child from receiving red meat, green vegetables, eggs, and bread (which are the main sources of iron). Older infants and toddlers are most at risk.

(iv) Children who suffer from chronic malabsorption who fail to absorb iron.

(v) Adolescent girls who are undergoing a phase of rapid growth at a time when they are also losing blood from menstruation.

Other deficiency anaemias are uncommon. Folic acid deficiency in British children may be seen in malabsorption syndromes. Pernicious anaemia is extremely rare in children. Hypothyroidism and scurvy are associated with hypochromic anaemias which are corrected by treatment of the primary condition.

(b) *Bone marrow disturbance*

Infiltration. Leukaemia (p. 238) is the most important infiltrative disturbance which may present as anaemia. Secondary deposits from malignant tumours and lipidoses are less common.

Toxic damage. Chronic infection and renal insufficiency depress haemopoiesis. A large number of poisons may suppress the cellular elements of the marrow and cause an *aplastic anaemia.* These include drugs, e.g. chloramphenicol.

2 Excessive breakdown

Haemolytic anaemias are not as common as deficiency anaemias, but are important in childhood as some are specific to children and others cause their main problems in childhood. They are characterized by chronic or recurrent normochromic anaemia. While haemolysis is active there is usually a reticulocytosis, but there is sometimes marrow aplasia at the time of acute haemolysis. When the haemolysis is severe and sudden it is called a 'haemolytic crisis'; jaundice, dark urine and dark stools are likely. Splenomegaly is a feature of chronic cases.

The main cause for the haemolysis may be an abnormality of the red blood cell, or an abnormal factor in the circulation.

(a) Cellular abnormalities

These can be conveniently grouped according to the way in which the abnormality is identified either by red cell shape, enzyme abnormality, or abnormal haemoglobin.

(i) Red cell shape. The most important abnormality is *hereditary spherocytosis* (acholuric jaundice) in which the red cells are fragile spherocytes and haemolyse easily. It is inherited as a dominant characteristic, but one-third of those affected have a negative family history.

(ii) Enzyme defect. The commonest defect is *glucose-6-phosphate dehydrogenase* (G6PD) *deficiency*. It is rare in Britain except in persons of Mediterranean, African or Chinese origin. Sex-linked recessive inheritance occurs. Affected children are susceptible to certain chemicals which cause haemolysis in them, but not in normal people. The list of possible chemicals is long, but most children with G6PD deficiency are harmed by only a few of them. PAS, primaquine and analine derivatives are particularly frequent pathogenic agents. Some of the children develop haemolysis after eating the bean or inhaling the pollen of the Fava bean (a type of broad bean); this is called *favism*.

(iii) *Haemoglobinopathies*. The synthesis of haemoglobin is under genetic control. Some abnormal genes interfere with the production of entire globin chains so that the affected person lacks normal haemoglobin (e.g. β-thalassaemia). Other abnormal genes result in the substitution of an abnormal amino acid in the globin chain, so producing an abnormal haemoglobin (e.g. HbS). These two examples are the most important haemoglobinopathies. Children with *thalassaemia* have a persistent preponderance of HbF and a deficiency of HbA. It is inherited by autosomal recessive genes and occurs in a broad equatorial belt extending from the Mediterranean countries through India to the Far East. The Mediterranean form is usually β-thalassaemia; α-thalassaemia, which is more severe and a common cause of neonatal death, occurs mainly in the Far East. In the United Kingdom most affected people have originated either from Cyprus or from the Indian subcontinent. Those with the heterozygous state have thalassaemia minor, and are asymptomatic or have a mild anaemia. Their red cells contain up to 20% HbF. Those with the homozygous state, thalassaemia major (Cooley's anaemia) develop severe haemolysis and anaemia in infancy. The children grow poorly and develop massive hepatosplenomegaly. Hyperplasia of the bone marrow leads to thickened skull bones. The best chance of survival for the child entails frequent blood transfusions, regular desferrioxamine therapy to reduce dangers of iron overload and folic acid supplement.

Sickle-cell disease occurs in the Negro races. HbS is present in place of HbA. At low oxygen tensions the cell becomes crescent or sickle-shaped and is likely to haemolyse. The heterozygotes have about 30% HbS, may show sickling, but are usually symptomless. The homozygotes develop recurrent episodes of haemolysis during infancy. In addition to the problems of haemolytic and aplastic episodes which occur in any haemolytic anaemia, those with sickle-cell disease also may develop intravascular thromboses. The thrombotic episodes cause local pain in the abdomen, bones and joints. The abdominal pain is commonly severe with signs resembling an acute abdominal emergency together with fever and leucocytosis. Treatment is symptomatic, and the prognosis poor; many die in late childhood or early adult life from infections, cardiac failure, or thrombotic episodes.

(b) *Extracellular abnormalities*

Antibodies causing premature destruction of the red cell are usually associated with a positive Coombs' test. Apart from haemolytic disease of the newborn (p. 35), circulating factors causing haemolysis are not common in childhood.

Haemolytic anaemia may occur secondary to malignancy or lupus erythematosus (rare in childhood) or as a complication of severe poisoning or infection.

3 Blood loss

Hidden blood loss is not common in childhood, peptic ulcers and gastrointestinal malignancy being rare. Gastrointestinal bleeding from a Meckel's diverticulum or a hiatus hernia is more likely to present with overt bleeding than unexplained anaemia.

COAGULATION DISORDERS

Haemophilia

Most cases (haemophilia A) are caused by deficiency of plasma factor VIII. A minority are caused by deficiency of factor IX (Christmas disease or haemophilia B). Both are cause by sex-linked recessive genes, so that half the sons of asymptomatic female carriers are affected. The condition usually presents during the second or third year of life, with bleeding following a trivial injury. Bleeding into soft tissues or into joints is particularly common. The haemarthroses particularly involving the knees are one of the major problems of haemophilia; recurrent haemarthrosis leads to permanent joint damage and chronic disability. The blood shows a prolonged clotting time and partial thromboplastin time; specific assay of the relevant coagulation factors is then performed to identify the precise abnormality.

Treatment of bleeding episodes consists of the intravenous injection of specially prepared concentrates of the deficient factor. This stops the bleeding, but transfusion may be needed to replace blood loss. Haemarthroses require careful orthopaedic management. One of the most difficult problems is in protecting the child from trauma, by special schooling and forbidding certain activities, and yet allowing the child to lead an enjoyable and profitable life. Regular prophylactic dental care is important and haemorrhage after dental extraction is avoided by admitting the child to hospital for factor replacement to cover the time of the extraction and the succeeding 2 days. Haemophilia usually becomes less severe as adult life is reached. Regional centres have been established to provide skilled co-ordinated care for haemophiliacs. One of their functions is to provide a service for the detection of women who carry the abnormal gene.

Thrombocytopenia

Thrombocytopenia may be a feature of several systemic diseases as well as infiltrative diseases of the bone marrow and marrow aplasia.

However, the most common thrombocytopenic purpura of childhood is *idiopathic thrombocytopenic purpura* (*ITP*), which occurs in healthy schoolchildren and is associated with a normal or near normal bone marrow which contains an excess of immature megakaryocytes. The onset is acute, often occurring 1–3 weeks after an upper respiratory tract infection. A widespread petechial rash appears, developing into small purpuric spots (purpuric spots do not fade when pressed). There may be bleeding from the nose or into the mucous membranes. Apart from the signs of bleeding there are no other abnormal signs, and the haemoglobin and white cell count are normal. The platelet count is low, usually below $30 \times 10^9/l$. During the onset period severe bleeding may occur, but generally the outcome is good. 75% of children have made a complete recovery within one month of onset and have no further trouble. Transfusions of platelets and blood may be needed at onset. Corticosteroids, given in large doses, reduce the risk of massive haemorrhage and accelerate the natural recovery in most children. Splenectomy is reserved for the small minority who have persistent or recurrent thrombocytopenia. Other causes of purpura are shown in Table 14.

Disseminated intravascular coagulation (DIC, consumption coagulopathy, fibrinolysis)

This syndrome is becoming increasingly recognised as an important cause of bleeding and purpura. It is convenient (though an oversimplification) to consider that intravascular coagulation uses up platelets and other factors, causing overt bleeding elsewhere; and that as the circu-

Table 14. The main causes of purpura in childhood

Platelet count low (thrombocytopenia)	Platelet count normal
Idiopathic thrombocytopenic purpura	Henoch–Schönlein syndrome (p. 197)
Leukaemia (p. 238)	Septicaemia (particularly meningococcal)
Toxic effect of drugs	Common infectious illnesses and viraemia

lating blood is forced through the intravascular clots some of the red cells are damaged, become fragmented and haemolyse. Therefore, the syndrome is associated with bleeding and a haemolytic anaemia, and may be diagnosed by the presence of fragmented red cells, thrombocytopenia and deficiency of coagulation factors. In the neonate it occurs as a result of severe anoxia or massive infection. In older children it may be associated with septicaemia, cyanotic congenital heart disease and vasculitis.

Further reading

Hardisty R. M. and Weatherall D. G. *Blood and its Disorders.* Blackwell Scientific Publications.

Willoughby M. L. N. *Paediatric Haematology.* Churchill-Livingstone.

Chapter 18

Malignant Disease

Malignant disease is the second most frequent cause of death between the ages of 1 and 15 years. Accidents are the commonest cause of death. Although malignancy is an important cause of death, it is nevertheless uncommon—only 1200 newly diagnosed cases occur in the United Kingdom annually out of a childhood population of approximately 12·5 millions.

Malignancy is not only less common than in adults, it is also different in origin and course. The epithelial malignancies of adult life, carcinomata of respiratory, gastrointestinal and reproductive tracts, are rarely seen in childhood. The commonest malignancies of childhood are those of the reticuloendothelial system: leukaemia and lymphoma. These are followed in order of frequency by brain tumours and then by primitive blast cell tumours and sarcomata of the kidney (Wilms' tumour), adrenal (neuroblastoma) and muscle tissue (rhabdomyosarcoma). Childhood tumours are relatively more malignant, disseminating early but responding well to therapy in most instances.

Leukaemia

This is nearly always acute lymphoblastic in type. It is commoner in boys and the peak age of onset is from 2 to 5 years. The presentation is likely to result from anaemia causing pallor and lethargy, or from thrombocytopenia causing purpura and bleeding. Fever is common and leukaemic deposits in the bones may cause limb pain. Lymphadenopathy, hepatomegaly and splenomegaly are variable, and frequently not present at onset.

Although the diagnosis must be confirmed by bone marrow examination, it is usually possible to make a presumptive diagnosis from examination of the peripheral blood; anaemia and thrombocytopenia are associated with lymphoblast cells. The total white count is more often normal or decreased than raised at onset. Subsequently leucocytosis may occur.

Initial treatment consists of induction of remission with vincristine, asparaginase and prednisolone combined with supportive therapy in the form of blood or platelet concentrates and antibiotics. 95% of children will achieve a remission within one month and be active and happy by then.

Because of the frequency with which meningeal leukaemia occurred in such treated children, it is now mandatory to follow the initial treatment with prophylactic irradiation of the central nervous system and then to maintain remission using either intermittent or continuous chemotherapy for 2–3 years.

The main results of modern aggressive therapy are that the duration of the first remission has increased greatly and CNS involvement has become less common. The mean length of survival is 5 years, and there are many individuals alive over 10 years from onset.

Lymphomas

These diseases are classified into Hodgkin's disease and non-Hodgkin's lymphoma. Each of these has several recognisable histological subdivisions but for treatment purposes only the two major categories need be considered. Hodgkin's disease is treated with radiotherapy and/or chemotherapy following careful evaluation of the extent of the disease. The prognosis is good. Non-Hodgkin's lymphoma is almost always generalised. It must be treated with intensive multiple drug chemotherapy and has a poor prognosis at present.

Central nervous system tumours

These are most commonly gliomas, either astrocytomas or medulloblastomas. They are mainly situated infratentorially and present with cerebellar signs (ataxia, incoordination, nystagmus) or raised intracranial pressure. In the young child the raised intracranial pressure will cause head enlargement and a bulging fontanelle, whilst in the older child with fused cranial sutures, pain and vomiting will be earlier symptoms. Papilloedema is an important early sign. 'Scanning' by computer-assisted tomography is proving as useful a diagnostic tool in children as in adults, though younger children may need a general anaesthetic to be sufficiently still for the test.

The treatment is primarily surgical; radiotherapy is used to eliminate any residual disease. The prognosis for benign cerebellar astrocytoma is good whilst that for the malignant medulloblastoma is poor.

Neuroblastoma

This is a malignant tumour arising from the sympathetic nervous tissue. It commonly arises from the adrenal gland but can arise in cervical, thoracic or lumbar sympathetic chains. The tumour presents as an abdominal mass most commonly, but early metastasis (to bone, liver and skin), is the rule, and these may be the presenting signs. An increased output of catecholamine degradation products (e.g. vanillylmandelic acid, HMMA) is usually present in the urine. The outlook is poor, except for some children under 1 year of age.

Wilms' tumour (nephroblastoma)

Nephroblastomas are embryonic renal tumours which usually present as a unilateral abdominal mass early in childhood. Microscopic haematuria occurs in up to a third of cases, but macroscopic haematuria is rare. Intravenous urogram shows a distorted kidney. Treatment often achieves complete cure.

Rhabdomyosarcoma

This tumour of striated muscle occurs in many different sites, but commonly is found in the genitourinary tract, the posterior abdominal wall, the nasopharynx or on the extremities.

TREATMENT OF CHILDHOOD MALIGNANCY

Specific treatment of childhood tumours is similar to that of adults. At one time surgery offered the best chance of cure, but it often had to be massive surgery leaving a child suffering from its mutilation. Increasingly irradiation and chemotherapy, singly or in combination, are becoming the mainstays of treatment. They too have potential snags: illness, disease and possible growth suppression from irradiation, and side-effects from the chemotherapy.

The social and psychological effects of malignant disease are considerable, particularly when superimposed on a child who may already be suffering from local or general symptoms from the tumour itself (usually most marked with CNS involvement). Every effort is made to keep the child out of hospital and leading a normal life at home and school. Many children with advanced disease can be treated on an outpatient basis providing there is good organisation and flexible, sympathetic staff. The best results are achieved when the child is treated in a specialised centre in which a multidisciplinary team is available to offer total care to the child and family.

Further reading

Jones P. G. and Campbell P. E. *Tumours of Infancy and Childhood.* Blackwell Scientific Publications.

Chapter 19

Endocrine and Metabolic Disorders

The essential difference between endocrine function in children and in adults is its importance in relation to physical and mental development. The relationships between the various glands, the controlling role of the pituitary, and the feed-back mechanisms, are established in pre-natal life. This chapter is not intended as a comprehensive catalogue of all the endocrine diseases that can occur in children, but as an indication of those which are most important in childhood or which differ significantly in their presentation or management in children.

Hypothyroidism

Normal thyroid function is necessary for normal physical and mental growth. Congenital absence of functional thyroid tissue causes *cretinism* which in turn leads to dwarfing and mental deficiency unless promptly recognized and treated. Lesser degrees of hypothyroidism may develop at any time during childhood, and may present as short stature.

A cretin is not recognizable as such at birth, but suspicions may first be aroused by prolonged physiological jaundice, coming on at the usual time (2nd or 3rd day) but lasting for 2, 3 or even 4 weeks. In the absence of this clue all may appear well for a few weeks, after which lethargy, difficulty with feeding, constipation, enlargement of the tongue, and umbilical hernia become noticeable. The cry may be deep and throaty. Early diagnosis is so important that there should never be the slightest hesitation in investigating a baby on suspicion. The facial appearance is characteristic to the trained eye (Fig. 59). The most helpful tests are estimation of plasma thyroxine

Fig. 59. A cretin aged 4 weeks. Compare with Fig. 60.

(T4) and TSH, and X-ray of relevant epiphyses which will show marked delay. In young babies the knee is more informative than the wrist. Tests using radioactive materials are not usually necessary, but the diagnosis must be established beyond doubt as it needs lifelong treatment. Treatment is with thyroxine starting with a small dose (e.g. 0·05 mg daily) and subsequently adjusting this according to the clinical response and periodic assessment of epiphyseal development. Excessive dosage will cause symptoms of thyrotoxicosis and accelerated epiphyseal development. If treatment is started within 2 or 3 months of birth and regularly maintained, there is a good chance of achieving normal physical and mental growth. The longer the delay, the poorer the prospects for mental development. Because of the difficulty of early diagnosis and the tragic consequences of delay, universal screening of newborns is being introduced, estimating T_4 and/or TSH on a filter paper blood spot.

Acquired hypothyroidism inhibits physical growth but

Fig. 60. A cretin aged 4 months. She has coarse features, dry mottled skin, scanty hair and an umbilical hernia.

may not affect school progress. It may be of thyroid or pituitary origin, and autoantibodies are sometimes present.

Goitre

Goitre is not common in childhood except in areas where it is endemic. A baby may be born with a goitre if the mother has taken antithyroid drugs (including iodides) during pregnancy. Goitre with thyrotoxicosis occurs rarely in childhood. In goitrous cretinism there is a metabolic block in the synthesis of thyroid hormone due to an autosomal recessive gene: the goitre takes a few years to develop. Some enlargement of the thyroid gland in adolescent girls is very common. Thyroid function is usually normal, but there may be temporary deficiency.

Diabetes mellitus

Diabetes in children is always of the ketotic, insulin-dependent variety, and diabetic children are almost always thin when first diagnosed. They usually present with a short history of polyuria, thirst and weight loss, or in pre-coma. There may be a family history of diabetes. The diagnosis is confirmed by demonstrating glucose and ketones in the urine and a high blood glucose level. The management of diabetes and diabetic coma in children is based on the same principles that apply to adult insulin-dependent diabetes. The following points are particularly relevant to children.

1   Carbohydrate intake must be carefully regulated, but the total calorie intake must be sufficient to maintain normal growth and to allow normal physical activities.

2   The child must learn to manage his own disease as soon as possible. Urine testing is now very simple, and an intelligent 7-year-old can inject his own insulin under supervision. All diabetic children should experience hypoglycaemia so that they can recognize it and know what to do about it.

3   The family must be helped to take diabetes in their stride so that it does not interfere with a normal way of life. Membership of the British Diabetic Association is helpful.

4   Diabetes in children is less stable than in adults. Periods of glycosuria are almost inevitable if hypoglycaemia is to be avoided. Insulin dosage often has to be reduced after the disease has first been brought under control.

5   Depression is common in diabetic adolescents.

The adrenal glands

Disorders of the adrenal gland are uncommon in children. The least rare is the adrenogenital syndrome. Total adrenocortical insufficiency (Addison's disease) is very rare. Adrenal cortical tumours may secrete androgens or oestrogens, with consequent appearance of the corresponding secondary sexual characteristics. Excess secretion of glucocorticoids and mineralocorticoids produces the clinical picture of Cushing's syndrome and may result from adenoma, carcinoma or hyperplasia of the adrenals.

The adrenogenital syndrome

This results from a metabolic block in the synthesis of hydrocortisone, the enzyme defect occurring in individuals homozygous for an autosomal recessive gene. The fetal adrenal normally secretes hydrocortisone, and the pituitary–adrenal axis is functional in prenatal life. This disorder therefore has its origins before birth. Hydrocortisone deficiency causes increased production of ACTH by the pituitary. This causes adrenal hyperplasia and excessive production of androgens. The affected female is therefore born with an enlarged clitoris, and often labial fusion. The genitalia of affected boys look normal at birth. Many affected children lack mineralocorticoids and early in life (often about the 2nd week) develop symptoms of salt loss—vomiting, dehydration, and collapse. This is lethal if not recognized and treated. In boys who are not salt-losers, diagnosis is likely to be delayed until is is recognized that both physical and sexual development are advancing with excessive speed (infant Hercules). Excessive androgens cause precocious pseudopuberty, advanced bone growth and advanced epiphyseal development. In untreated cases epiphyseal fusion occurs very early and ultimate stature is therefore small.

In cases presenting as intersex, buccal smear and chromosome studies will show a normal female pattern. The diagnosis is confirmed by finding raised levels of androgen metabolites and hydrocortisone precursors (17-oxosteroids and pregnanetriol) in urine. Lowered serum sodium and chloride, with raised potassium levels, may be demonstrated in salt-losers. Some affected children are hypertensive.

Treatment is essentially the oral replacement of missing hormones. Cortisone or prednisolone is required by all patients, with additional fludrocortisone for the salt-losers. Precise dosage and spacing of doses is important. Inadequate control will permit excessive growth and subsequent stunting: excess steroids will stunt growth. Treatment must be lifelong, with increased dosage at times of stress. Plastic surgery may be required before school age to correct labial fusion or to recess a large clitoris.

Cushing's syndrome

This is most commonly seen in children who have been treated with steroids for long periods (Fig. 61). The face is fat and plethoric and there is excess facial hair. The whole body is obese and there are striae, especially on the

Fig. 61. Cushing's syndrome from prolonged corticosteroid therapy. The face is round, hirsute and plethoric.

abdomen. There may be hypertension or glycosuria. The effect of endogenous steroids on growth is variable, but a common hazard of long-term steroid administration is growth retardation (see p. 259).

Pituitary disorders

Pituitary dwarfism is described on page 55.

Diabetes insipidus

This is a rare disease, resulting from either failure of the hypothalamus to produce sufficient antidiuretic hormone (ADH) or failure of the renal tubule to respond to it (nephrogenic diabetes insipidus). In either case there is marked thirst and the passage of large volumes of almost colourless urine of low specific gravity and osmolality. There is a constant danger of serious water depletion, especially in hot weather, and growth is retarded. ADH deficiency may result from a variety of intracranial disorders, including tumours, cysts, vascular accidents, and meningitis. It may also result from an isolated hormone deficiency, genetically determined. In ADH-deficient cases, desmopressin or pitressin can be given by injection, or intranasally. Nephrogenic diabetes insipidus is caused by a sex-linked gene and therefore occurs only in males.

The gonads

Gonadal dysgenesis and testicular feminisation are dealt with elsewhere (p. 66) as are undescended testicles (p. 67). Gonadal tumours are fortunately very rare. They may secrete androgens or oestrogens, leading to masculinisation or feminisation. Testicular tumours may be very small and difficult to detect.

INBORN ERRORS OF METABOLISM

This term was originally coined by Garrod to embrace three disorders but the list has now grown to many hundreds. Most are genetically determined, usually by autosomal recessive genes, and most are extremely rare. In some, the metabolic block leads to deficiency of metabolites beyond the block and accumulation of precursors and their metabolites. Many conditions of this type lead to mental deficiency unless effective treatment can be instituted early. In others the outstanding feature is failure of reabsorption by the renal tubules of one or more substances, usually with profound metabolic consequences. Reference will only be made to a small number of conditions which illustrate general principles.

Phenylketonuria

In this disorder, which affects about 1 in 10–20 000 children born, deficiency of phenylalanine hydroxylase interferes with the conversion of phenylalanine to tyrosine. Phenylalanine levels in the blood and tissues rise, and abnormal metabolites (phenylketones) are excreted in the urine. The most serious consequence is mental defect, but there is also physical stunting, and in some cases eczema or convulsions in early infancy. The symptoms appear to be caused, at least predominantly, by the accumulation of phenylalanine and its derivatives rather than to deficiency of tyrosine. Hence, treatment by the controlled restriction of phenylalanine in the diet is helpful, and if started before the age of 2 months ensures normal development. It is for this reason that programmes of population screening for the disease have been instituted in many countries. The most widely used screening procedure at present is the Guthrie test, which uses a phenylalanine-dependent strain of *Bacillus subtilis* as a biological indicator of serum phenylalanine concentration. It must be emphasised that this is a screening test designed to detect phenylalanine levels above 250 μmol/l: the diagnosis of phenylketonuria requires further biochemical testing of blood and urine. The baby should be receiving a satisfactory protein intake at the time of the test, otherwise a false-negative result may occur.

Dietetic management is difficult. It requires careful biochemical control so that the serum phenylalanine is maintained within acceptable limits. Some of the amino-acid foods are not very palatable, and as the children get older it may be difficult to control what they eat. Some relaxation of dietary control can be allowed after 10 years of age, but if a normal diet is resumed too soon behaviour disorders are common. Adult phenylketonuric women have given birth to mentally retarded (though not phenylketonuric) children, presumably because of damage to the fetal brain by high levels of phenylalanine crossing the placenta. Dietetic restrictions should therefore be resumed before conception and throughout pregnancy.

The disorder is caused by an autosomal recessive gene. There is therefore a 25% risk of recurrence in siblings. Carriers can be detected with a reasonable degree of accuracy by a phenylalanine loading test.

Galactosaemia

Although some centres screen all infants for galactosaemia, it is not widely practised because affected babies become ill almost as soon as they begin to drink milk. A deficiency of galactose-1-phosphate-uridyl-transferase leads to accumulation of galactose in the blood and tissues and its excretion in the urine. Early symptoms are vomiting, weight loss, jaundice and hepatomegaly. Galactose (a reducing sugar) appears in the urine, provided sufficient milk feeds have been taken and retained. Hypoglycaemia may also be evident, and untreated survivors later show mental defect, cataract and cirrhosis of the liver, with hepatoma developing in some. Treatment is by the exclusion of lactose from the diet. The response is good for physical growth, less good for intellectual growth.

Babies with funny smells

Occasionally a newborn baby is noted, usually by the nursing staff, to smell strange. Some of these babies prove to have inborn errors of metabolism, the smell being due to abnormal substances in the urine. Phenylketonurics are said to have a characteristic smell, and several disorders in the group are named after the smell, e.g., maple syrup urine disease, oast-house disease, and even the odour-of-sweaty-feet syndrome. The observation of a strange smell from a baby should never be ignored.

RENAL TUBULAR DEFECTS

In this group of disorders, also genetically determined, there is failure of tubular reabsorption of one or more essential substances. Reference is made on page 248 to nephrogenic diabetes insipidus, which is a defect of tubular reabsorption of water. Phosphate, bicarbonate, glucose and amino-acids are lost in other disorders.

Vitamin D-resistant rickets

This results from tubular loss of phosphate and is a feature of several rare disorders. It usually presents with bowing of the legs in the second year of life.

It will respond to large doses of vitamin D (25–100 000 units daily), but excessive dosage will lead to nephrocalcinosis and arterial calcification. Management is therefore difficult.

In *cystinosis*, cystine is stored in the tissues, there is vomiting, failure to thrive, rickets, and eventual renal failure. Cystine crystals may be demonstrated in bone marrow and by slit-lamp examination in the cornea. (This should not be confused with *cystinuria* in which there is tubular loss of cystine, sometimes with the formation of cystine stones).

HYPOGLYCAEMIA

Hypoglycaemia is not a disease but a symptom. The maintenance of normal blood glucose levels depends upon the ingestion, absorption and metabolism of carbohydrates, and normal levels of insulin, glucocorticoids and other hormones. A wide variety of diseases may therefore be associated with hypoglycaemia. Early symptoms include hunger, irritability, pallor, sweating and tachycardia. Later symptoms include convulsions and coma. Some symptoms are probably directly due to low tissue glucose levels, others to the secretion of adrenalin which normally ensues.

Hypoglycaemia in the newborn is most often seen in low birthweight babies (especially the light-for-dates) and in the infants of diabetic mothers (p. 32). Symptomatic hypoglycaemia is only exceptionally seen in starvation or malabsorption states, although blood glucose levels may be moderately low, and glucose tolerance curves flat. Amongst metabolic disorders, hypoglycaemia is a feature of galactosaemia and some types of glycogen storage disease. It may also occur during the prediabetic phase of diabetes mellitus in children. Insulin overdosage is, of course, the commonest cause of hypoglycaemia. Insulinoma is very rare.

A few infants develop hypoglycaemia after ingestion of leucine, iso-leucine or valine. The attacks therefore tend to be postprandial. Children with hypopituitarism from any cause may have hypoglycaemic episodes and are unduly sensitive to insulin. *Ketotic hypoglycaemia* occurs in thin children under 5 years, especially boys. Symptoms occur chiefly in the mornings and are relieved by glucose. Prolonged fasting usually fails to precipitate an attack, but a ketogenic diet may do so. Spontaneous remission occurs by 10 years.

Repeated hypoglycaemic fits may lead to brain damage and must therefore be treated vigorously. Emergency treatment consists of the intravenous injection of 50% glucose solution, which will rapidly stop fits and restore consciousness. The underlying cause must be sought and, if possible, treated. If the fundamental cause cannot be treated, diazoxide, steroids or ACTH may be helpful.

Further reading

Hubble D. *Paediatric Endocrinology*. Blackwell Scientific Publications.
Wilkins L. *Endocrine Disorders in Childhood*. Thomas, Illinois.
Sinclair L. *Metabolic Disease in Childhood*. Blackwell Scientific Publications.

Chapter 20

Therapeutics

Therapeutics is not to be regarded as synonymous with the prescription of drugs. Drugs often have an important role, but therapy includes all measures taken to relieve symptoms and to hasten recovery. In the management of medical (as distinct from surgical) conditions in children, the doctor's function is almost entirely advisory, the therapy being carried out largely by the mother at home or by nurses in hospital. Some problems need the help of specialized therapists (e.g. physiotherapists, speech therapists, occupational therapists).

GENERAL MEASURES

In any acute illness advice needs to be given about some basic aspects of management, and a worried mother caring for a sick child at home will appreciate clear guidance.

1 *Rest.* A child who feels ill will want to rest: one who feels well will not. There are very few indications for trying to enforce rest. Active disease of the heart or lungs may restrict activity, as will painful joints, but enforced inactivity will almost always do more harm than good. At home, the sofa or a comfortable chair downstairs with the TV set is more conducive to rest than bored isolation in the bedroom.

Hypoxic babies with heart or lung disease are often restless and may require sedation as well as oxygen.

2 *Temperature and humidity.* There is still a widespread fear that febrile children may suffer from chilling, and consequently parents switch on bedroom heaters and pile on blankets. Such measures can only help raise body temperature and increase discomfort and the risk of febrile convulsion in young children. Room temperature

should be comfortable (about 18°C, 65°F), preferably with an open window. High fever in a young child is an indication for active cooling by giving antipyretics, removing blankets, using fans and, if necessary, tepid sponging.

Dry air is irritating to an inflamed respiratory tract and may aggravate cough. Central heating often dries the air and this can be overcome by placing a reservoir of water by the radiator. Active humidification may give relief in laryngitis and is achieved more safely by cold humidity than by steam. High humidity can only be achieved in a tent. There is no evidence that humidification is helpful in chest infections. Even in cystic fibrosis, controlled trials have so far shown no advantage, even using ultrasonic nebulizers which produce very small droplets.

A sheltered corner of a sunny garden is a far better place than a bedroom for convalescence.

3   *Diet.* During acute illnesses, especially febrile illnesses, drinking is much more important than eating. The child should be encouraged to drink frequent small quantities of water, fruit juice or glucose drinks. A vomiting child should have a small drink after each vomit: some will return with the next vomit, but some will stay down. Fluid intake may need to be more accurately controlled and recorded in renal disease, and output should be recorded in renal disease and heart failure.

It does not matter if a sick child eats little or nothing for a few days. Parents should be told that the lost weight will soon be regained. Appetite is a good guide, and a little of what the child fancies will probably do good. Returning appetite is a good sign of returning health. In some renal disorders, diabetes mellitus, coeliac disease and inborn errors of metabolism, more strictly controlled diets are needed.

4   *Isolation.* Children with infectious diseases nursed at home do not necessarily need to be isolated. Measles and chicken pox are highly infectious before the spots appear, and siblings are probably already infected when the rash develops. With rubella, the risk to pregnant women must be remembered. Infective hepatitis is unpleasant, especially in adults. Barrier nursing with disinfection of excreta is advisable at home as in hospital.

254   5   *Schoolwork.* To miss any substantial time from school

may set back a child's educational progress, especially if this happens around the time of crucial examinations. In most hospitals teachers are made available by education authorities to work on children's wards. At home, teachers are usually glad to provide schoolwork and will sometimes call in to help with problems. For children confined to their homes for long periods, regular home teaching may be provided. Children who have been ill should be allowed back to school as soon as possible, if necessary on a part-time basis initially, but physical activities (games and PE) may need to be postponed for longer.

DRUGS

When these general points have been attended to, more often than not it will be appropriate to prescribe one or more drugs. In spite of the enormous number of drugs and compounds available, the wise doctor will confine his prescribing to a relatively small number of drugs with which he is familiar. The newest drug is not necessarily the best, and is certainly the one of which there is least experience. An old remedy is not necessarily a bad one. Experienced doctors find that they can treat all but the most obscure conditions with fewer than fifty drugs.

The prescription of a drug for a patient is often done with little thought at all, but if medicine is to be practised at its best, it demands a 10-point catechism.

1 *Is a drug necessary?* Am I treating a symptom or the underlying disease, or am I prescribing a placebo to make anxious parents or myself feel better? Is this a virus infection, because if so I might be wiser to avoid antibiotics?

2 *If so, which one?* If an antibiotic, what organisms are likely to be involved and what will be effective against them? What drug has the best chance of doing good without doing harm? Prefer a familiar drug to an unfamiliar. Other things being equal, economize. The use of official names may save money.

3 *Which preparation shall I use?* Try to find something palatable for young children. Don't order capsules for babies unless it is permissible to put the contents in a

spoon. Some young children prefer tablets: some older ones prefer medicines. Ask the mother.

4   *What route of administration?* Don't give injections if they can be avoided, *but* they may be necessary if the child is vomiting or if it is necessary to achieve high tissue levels quickly. If there is peripheral circulatory failure, drugs given by intramuscular injection may be absorbed slowly. If there is serious infection (meningitis, septicaemia) give antibiotics intravenously to begin with.

5   *How much, how often, for how long?* There is no infallible formula for calculating dosage for children. The younger the child, the more critical the dose (especially the newborn baby). There is a big margin of safety for some drugs, but very little for others, such as digoxin. Therefore, put the child's age or date of birth on the prescription. This gives the pharmacist a chance to check the dose. Frequency of administration depends on the duration of action of the drug. Do not disturb sleep unnecessarily. Arrange an infant's drug schedule to fit in with the feeding schedule (i.e. avoid ordering 6-hourly drugs and 4-hourly feeds). Remember to specify the duration of treatment.

6   *Is the drug compatible with the patient?* Is there any history of drug allergy or other untoward reaction? Has he any disorder which limits the use of any drugs (e.g. glucose-6-phosphate dehydrogenase deficiency).

7   *Is the drug compatible with other drugs?* If two or more drugs are being given, ensure that they do not inhibit or potentiate one another. Be especially careful of mixing drugs for intravenous administration.

8   *Have I written the prescription legibly?*

9   *Have I given any necessary instructions about the administration of the drug or its storage?*

10   *Have I given any necessary warning* of side effects, whether harmless (e.g. dark stools with iron) or serious?

A general indication of the drugs appropriate for the treatment of common conditions will be found in the other chapters of this book, but some comments on common prescribing problems are included here. In most clinical situations there is no one line of treatment that is undoubtedly superior to all others and you may therefore meet a bewildering variety of therapeutic approaches amongst your medical teachers. Sometimes you may meet direct conflict, one teacher advising you never to do something that another habitually does. Have courage and ask the reason why.

Prescribing for the newborn

Very few drugs are needed for the treatment of neonatal disease, and some are positively harmful. Many of the metabolic functions of the liver and the excretory capacity of the kidneys take a week or so to develop fully. During this time very high blood levels of drugs may be achieved on relatively low dosage. This is especially true of the pre-term infant. Chloramphenicol, sulphonamides, tetracyclines, lincomycin and novobiocin should be avoided altogether. Serious infections at this age are usually caused by gram-negative bacteria (chiefly *E. coli*) and are best treated with gentamicin combined with ampicillin *or* penicillin. Naloxone (0·01 mg/kg i.m.) is an antidote to morphine, pethidine and pentazocine. Stimulants such as ethamivan are sometimes used in infants with respiratory depression. Irritability and convulsions due to cerebral problems may be controlled with phenobarbitone or chloral hydrate, but if due to metabolic disturbances (e.g. hypoglycaemia) appropriate correction must be made.

Oxygen is a powerful therapeutic weapon for good or ill. In the severely asphyxiated newborn, endotracheal oxygen is the most pressing need. In respiratory and some cardiac problems the intelligent use of oxygen is crucial. Excessive concentrations of oxygen can damage the eyes, the brain and the lungs. Monitoring of blood gases is therefore essential.

Digoxin must always be used with care, especially in the newborn and most of all in the pre-term infant. The margin between therapeutic and toxic doses is narrow and in the event of overdosage there is no effective antidote. Calculate the dose with care and watch hawk-eyed for early signs of toxicity.

Iron and vitamin supplements are needed by all pre-term babies. It is not *necessary* to start them before 6 weeks, and little iron is absorbed before this time, but it is *convenient* to start them before the baby is discharged home.

Antibiotics

If there are infections in paradise the causative organism will be known every time and there will be available an antibiotic which kills that organism and no others. In this life we must make an intelligent guess at the organism (the laboratory may give us help after a day or two) and decide what chemotherapy is appropriate. If the infection is certainly or probably viral (measles, influenza, laryngitis) antibiotics are not needed. The notion of 'preventing secondary bacterial infection' is not valid in children. In some bacterial infections, especially bacillary dysentery, there is good evidence that antibiotics do harm. There may be genuine diagnostic uncertainties, as between bronchiolitis (viral) and bronchopneumonia (viral or bacterial) in infants.

If swabs or samples of urine, faeces, blood or CSF are needed for culture, take them before starting antibiotics. Swabs, unless of frank pus, need to be taken thoroughly, transported expeditiously and incubated promptly.

Some antibiotics cause diarrhoea, others (especially ampicillin) cause rashes. Such symptoms often settle in spite of continuation of the drug. Babies given broad-spectrum antibiotics often develop oral thrush (moniliasis). Tetracyclines should be avoided under the age of 7 years because they damage and discolour the teeth.

If an unnecessary antibiotic has been started, stop it as soon as possible.

Anticonvulsants

The drugs appropriate to the treatment of different forms of epilepsy are discussed in Chapter 6.

Phenobarbitone is often tolerated well by children but may make them hyperactive. Blood levels fall after the first week or two of treatment because the induction of liver enzymes leads to more rapid inactivation. If half the calculated dose is given for the first fortnight, early side-effects will be minimized. If facilities are available for determining serum levels, these provide a helpful indication of the adequacy of the dose and reliability of administration.

Sodium valproate, ethosuximide and carbamezapine

are relatively free from side-effects. Phenytoin nearly always causes some gum hyperplasia which goes when the drug is stopped. Children taking it need good dental care. Hirsutism and ataxia are not uncommon. Rickets and megaloblastic anaemia (responsive to folates) occur infrequently.

Changes in drugs or in dosage for epileptic children should be made gradually. Push each drug to the limit of tolerance before abandoning it. Try to avoid giving several drugs simultaneously.

Sedatives and tranquillisers

It should only exceptionally be necessary to prescribe these drugs for children. The use of hypnotics for sleep disturbances is described on page 127. Tranquillisers are sometimes needed for children with behaviour disorders, but they should only be used as an adjunct to attempts to determine and influence the cause of the misbehaviour.

Steroids

Cortisone and its many relatives may be used either locally or systemically, for short- or long-term treatment.

Local steroids include many preparations for the treatment of skin conditions (e.g. betamethasone for eczema) and steroids for inhalation (e.g. beclamethasone for asthma). The quantities of steroid absorbed from these preparations appears to be minimal.

Short-term oral or parenteral steroids are valuable in the treatment of severe asthmatic attacks, overwhelming infections and allergic reactions. In this critical situation big doses should be given, but can soon be stopped.

Medium-term (a few weeks) oral steroids are used to induce remissions in leukaemia, the nephrotic syndrome and some autoimmune disorders. During treatment excessive weight gain, plethora and hirsutism commonly develop, but subside when treatment is stopped. More serious side effects are rare.

Long-term (months or years) oral steroids are rarely needed and often cause side effects, notably stunting of growth, except when they are being used as replacement therapy. This is specially so in very young children.

259

Regular checks of weight, height, blood pressure, urine (for diabetes), eyes (for cataract) and spine X-ray (for osteoporosis) should be made. Stunting of height may be reduced by giving intermittent (e.g. alternate day) steroids, or by using ACTH or tetracosactrin which must be injected. Single daily doses are best given in the morning to fit in with the normal circadian rhythm. Excessive weight gain can be prevented by calorie control.

After medium- and long-term therapy, steroid dosage should be reduced gradually. The normal pituitary response to stress may be impaired for some months thereafter, so steroid cover for operations, etc. is needed.

Salicylates

In paediatrics, salicylates are used either in modest dosage for a short period or in heroic doses for a longer period. The first is an effective way to relieve pains and reduce fever. If soluble aspirin is given in a sensible dose for not more than 2 or 3 days at a time, it is safe drug at any age.

In acute rheumatism (rheumatic fever) salicylates have a specific effect, but should be given in maximal dosage for maximal relief (see p. 196). They are also the drug of first choice for rheumatoid arthritis, and here again big doses may be necessary. In children with capillary or platelet defects salicylates should be avoided. Paracetamol may be used instead. Benorylate is a complex of paracetamol and salicylate which breaks down into its components in the body.

Further reading

Burland W. L. & Laurance B. M. (eds) *The Therapeutic Choice in Paediatrics.* Churchill-Livingstone.

Gellis S. S. and Kagan B. M. *Current Paediatric Therapy,* Saunders.

Wood B. S. B. *A Paediatric Vade-Mecum,* Lloyd-Luke.

Chapter 21

Immunity, Immunization and Specific Fevers

Most illness in childhood is infective, and an important activity in the early life of every individual is meeting and establishing immunity to a wide variety of infecting organisms. Immunological mechanisms in childhood are essentially the same as in adults but are not fully developed at birth. Cellular immunity is effective from birth: for the first 2 or 3 years of life, lymphocytes predominate over polymorphs in the circulating blood, but the total white cell count is relatively high (p. 230). Pus can be formed at any age. Humoral immunity is slower to develop. Maternal IgG is transferred across the placenta from early fetal life and in the full-term infant approximates to adult levels. This conveys passive immunity to a number of common infections, including measles, rubella and mumps. In contrast, the larger molecules of IgM do not cross the placenta and the neonate is therefore fully susceptible to bacterial infections including pertussis. The fetus is capable of making its own IgM in response to intrauterine infection, e.g. rubella, but synthesis of other immunoglobulins gets off to a rather sluggish start after birth. A reasonable level of humoral immunity is established by the age of 6–9 months (Fig. 62).

Pre-term babies have relatively low levels of circulating immunoglobulins, and are particularly susceptible to infection. Total immunoglobulin levels in all infants reach their lowest at about 3–4 months of age which is another susceptible period. In older children, recurrent infections are rarely due to immunological deficiencies. Poor social conditions and debilitating diseases such as cystic fibrosis or congenital heart disease may predispose to infection. Recurrent skin infections may be associated with nasal carriage of *Staph. pyogenes*, and recurrent

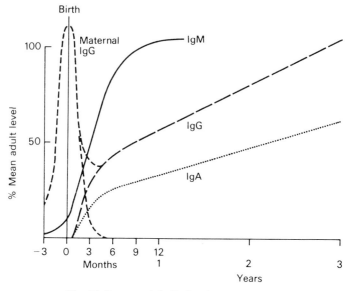

Fig. 62. Immunoglobulin levels in early life.

urinary infections with congenital anomalies of the renal tract or vesicoureteric reflux. Rarely, however, repeated infections, especially of the skin and lungs, may be due to some defect of the defence mechanisms. Cellular immunity may be impaired by deficiency of granulocytes (seen especially in children undergoing treatment with cytotoxic drugs) or by qualitative defects of the white cells, as in chronic granulomatous disease. Hypogammaglobulinaemia is encountered in a number of rare disorders.

IMMUNIZATION

As infectious diseases account for a large part of the mortality and morbidity of early childhood it is logical to institute whatever preventive measures are available. Table 15 shows the programme of immunization currently recommended for children in the U.K. In determining such a schedule, two basic decisions need to be made.

262

Table 15. Schedule of immunization procedures

Age	Prophylactic	Notes
Starting at 3 months	Diph/Tet/Pert and oral polio vaccine (first dose)	
	Diph/Tet/Pert and oral polio vaccine (second dose). Preferably after an interval of 6–8 weeks	
	Diph/Tet/Pert and oral polio vaccine (third dose). Preferably after an interval of 4–6 months	
During the second year of life	Measles vaccination. At least 3 weeks after 3rd dose of Triple/Polio vaccine	Live measles vaccine should not be given to children below the age of 15 months
At school entry	Diph/Tet and oral polio vaccine	These may be given earlier to children entering nursery schools, attending day nurseries or living in children's homes
Age 10–13 years	BCG vaccine	For tuberculin-negative children
Age 11–14 years	Rubella vaccine	For girls
On leaving school	Polio vaccine. Tetanus toxoid	

(1) Against what diseases should a child be protected? This requires a balance of the probabilities of him (a) catching it, (b) suffering death or disability from it, and (c) the dangers and effectiveness of the immunizing procedure. The more common and the more dangerous the disease, and the safer the immunization, the greater the need. (2) At what age should immunization be done? This depends upon the age of susceptibility of the child and the age at which he can best respond to the vaccine. There is

263

often a conflict here, as in the case of pertussis. The greatest danger of the disease is in the first 6 months of life, but the immunological response is relatively poor before 6 months of age. Immunizing procedures should be avoided in children who are not completely well and live vaccine should not be given to those who are immunologically depressed (from disease or drugs). Live vaccine viruses may be transmitted from person to person in a household: the risk to pregnant women must be remembered.

Diphtheria

This has become an excessively rare disease in Britain, whereas at the turn of the century it was a major cause of death in childhood. The continuance of this happy state depends upon continuing immunization of as many infants as possible. The toxoid scarcely ever causes any disturbance and there are no contraindications to its use in young children.

Tetanus

Tetanus is rare, but the mortality rate is still substantial and routine immunization is wise. Tetanus toxoid is safe and effective. This contrasts with anti-tetanus serum (ATS) which is prepared from horse serum and frequently causes reactions, some of which are serious and a few fatal. The value of ATS is limited because antibodies to it are rapidly developed and it is likely that any dose except the first received by an individual is rapidly inactivated. ATS should be reserved for the treatment of tetanus.

Pertussis

Pertussis vaccine, prepared from killed whooping cough bacilli, is the third component of triple vaccine and is the only one of the three to cause any disturbance of health. Minor reactions are common, restlessness, fever or transient screaming episodes coming on a few hours after the injection. They last a few hours. Occasionally the temperature rises high enough to cause a febrile convulsion. It has been suggested that pertussis vaccine may cause neurological damage. Recent studies suggest that this is a

264

very rare occurrence. Nevertheless it is recommended that it should not be given to infants with any evidence of disordered brain function (e.g. fits or cerebral palsy), with a family history of such conditions in close relatives, or to a child who has had a previous reaction to pertussis immunization.

Poliomyelitis

Poliomyelitis vaccine is usually given in the oral form (Sabin vaccine) which contains live virus. Side effects are practically unknown and the only contraindications are known sensitivity to penicillin, streptomycin, neomycin or polymyxin. It is highly effective.

Smallpox

In 1980 the world was officially declared free from smallpox. Vaccination against it is therefore no longer necessary, although a few sceptical countries continue to demand evidence of vaccination from visitors and immigrants.

Measles

Measles vaccination with a live attenuated vaccine is generally safe and effective. A mild measles-like illness may occur after the immunization. Hypersensitivity to egg protein, neomycin or polymyxin are contraindications. Simultaneous administration of human immunoglobulin is recommended if there is chronic disease or a family history of convulsions. Untreated active tuberculosis is a contraindication.

Rubella

This is not a danger except to the embryo. In Britain vaccination with a live attenuated rubella virus is recommended for girls aged 11–14 years, and to adult females and selected males who are shown to be non-immune. The duration of immunity is not yet known but is unlikely to be less than 10 years.

BCG

BCG vaccination gives substantial protection against tuberculosis (and leprosy). It is injected intradermally over the insertion of the deltoid muscle. After 3–6 weeks there is local erythema, induration and sometimes ulceration. The axillary glands may enlarge and be painful. The local signs go in 2–6 months. The use of BCG varies greatly in different countries: in some, BCG is given routinely to all infants. In Britain schoolchildren have a tuberculin test at the age of 10–12 years and the 90% who are tuberculin negative are subsequently given BCG. Babies are given BCG during the neonatal period if anyone in the immediate family has had TB.

DIAGNOSIS OF INFECTIONS

In children with unexplained fever and in some in whom a firm 'disease diagnosis' has been made (e.g. meningitis) it is often important to try to establish the responsible organism. This may be achieved by:
1 Identification of the organism
    (a) by microscopic techniques
    (b) by culture.
2 Demonstration of a rise of specific antibody titre.

Direct light microscopy of unstained material from body fluids (e.g. urine, CSF), pus and biopsy specimens, may reveal identifiable bacteria. Electron microscopy is more appropriate for viruses. Immunofluorescent techniques allow rapid, positive identification. Swabs should be taken thoroughly (especially throat swabs) and transported to the laboratory swiftly. Skin scrapings are needed to identify skin fungi. Blood cultures are best taken when fever is rising. Take all necessary bacteriological specimens before giving antibiotics, if possible. Material for virological culture must be put straight into transport medium.

Demonstration of a significant *rise* in antibody titre, whether bacterial (e.g. ASO) or viral, requires at least two specimens, one taken early in the illness, another 10 days–3 weeks later. A single convalescent sample showing a high antibody titre must be interpreted more cautiously.

SPECIFIC FEVERS

The main clinical features of the common infectious diseases of childhood together with their incubation periods and important complications are listed in Table 16. Infectivity is usually maximal in the prodromal stage and ends within a week of definitive signs appearing. The following paragraphs describe the aspects of these diseases which are important in childhood.

Measles (morbilli)

This usually presents with respiratory catarrh, misery, fever and a rash. Less frequent presentations include febrile convulsion and epistaxis. Sometimes the prodrome appears prolonged, with unexplained, intermittent fever. A prodromal rash, quite unlike a measles rash, may appear at about the time of appearance of Koplik's spots. Otitis media and bronchopneumonia are common complications: encephalitis affects about 1 in 1000 cases. In the absence of complications, antibiotics are not indicated.

Rubella (German measles)

Rubella may also present with epistaxis. In general the illness is very mild and there are virtually no complications. The arthralgia of the hands so common in adolescent and adult females does not affect children.

Chicken pox (varicella)

This is usually a mild disease. The differential diagnosis is from papular urticaria (p. 210) which, if scratched and infected, also presents papules, vesicles, pustules and scabs. However, the lesions in chicken pox are predominantly on the trunk, whilst papular urticaria is peripherally distributed. Complications are rare. Chicken pox encephalitis presents as ataxia a week or so after the rash has appeared; the prognosis is good.

Mumps

This is most commonly confused with cervical adenitis.

Table 16. Common infectious diseases

Disease	Incubation period (days)*	Main features	Important complications	Laboratory findings
Measles	7–*10*–12	Misery, fever, catarrh, cough, conjunctivitis; Koplik's spots; blotchy, red rash on face and trunk	Pneumonia Otitis media Encephalitis	Rise in antibody titre
Rubella	10–*18*–21	Upper respiratory catarrh; macular or erythematous rash, chiefly on trunk; cervical adenopathy	Virtually none in childhood Encephalitis very rare	Virus culture from stool or nose Rise in antibody titre
Chickenpox	10–*14*–21	Rash on trunk, perineum and scalp; papules, vesicles, pustules, scabs; fever at pustular stage	Conjunctival lesions Encephalitis	
Mumps	14–*18*–28	Parotitis, sometimes involvement of other salivary glands	Meningitis Pancreatitis Orchitis after puberty	Virus from saliva Rise in antibody titre Lymphocytosis
Whooping-cough	7–*10*–14	Upper respiratory catarrh; paroxysmal cough with vomiting. Modified greatly by immunization	Pneumonia Lobar collapse Convulsions Haemorrhage (nose, eyes, brain)	*B. pertussis* from cough plate or per-nasal swab Lymphocytosis + +
Scarlet fever	1–*3*–7	Tonsillitis (pharyngitis); diffuse, erythematous rash chiefly on trunk; sore, coated tongue; circumoral pallor	Otitis media Rheumatic fever Acute nephritis	Gp. A haem. strep. from throat Rise in ASO titre

* Outer figures = range, centred italic figure = usual

The exact location of the swelling, the fact that it is nearly always bilateral, the swelling of the orifice of the parotid ducts, and absence of any cause for cervical adenitis, should make the diagnosis clear. Mumps is the commonest cause of lymphocytic meningitis, and can occur without parotitis (p. 91). Pancreatitis and orchitis are rare before puberty. Rarely nerve deafness occurs.

Whooping-cough (pertussis)

Whooping-cough is a serious disease in the very young infant, and unpleasant at all ages. Babies with pertussis do not whoop, but the cough is paroxysmal and associated with vomiting. The cough is worse at night in children who are upright during the day. Severe spasms may lead to capillary rupture (which is common in the conjunctivae) or may lead to hypoxia sufficient to cause a convulsion. Lobar collapse is not uncommon and may lead to bronchiectasis if not detected and treated. Encephalopathy is rare. In children who have been immunized the disease tends to be mild, the whoop absent, and there may be no lymphocytosis: the diagnosis is then easily missed.

Scarlet fever (scarlatina)

This has become a rare disease since the introduction of penicillin.

Roseola infantum (exanthem subitum)

Roseola infantum is a mild disease of infants and young children, common outside hospital but rarely severe enough to need admission. Catarrhal symptoms and fever for 2 or 3 days are followed by the abrupt appearance of light red, discrete macules on the trunk. As the rash appears, the fever rapidly settles and the child is greatly improved. A few days later, the illness is over.

Glandular fever (infectious mononucleosis)

Glandular fever results from infection with Epstein–Barr virus, but a similar clinical picture may result from infection by several viruses or by *Toxoplasma gondii*. The onset is gradual, with malaise, anorexia and low-grade fever for 1–2 weeks, after which more specific signs may develop.

1 Lymphadenopathy—multiple, firm, discrete, non-tender glands especially in the neck. They never suppurate.

2 Splenomegaly.

3 Pharyngitis.

4 Rash in some cases, macular or urticarial. Ampicillin often causes a morbilliform rash.

5 Jaundice—resulting from an associated hepatitis or from enlarged glands in the porta hepatis.

6 Meningeal involvement, with headache, stiff neck, and raised cells and protein in the CSF.

In classical glandular fever the peripheral blood shows an increased number of mononuclear cells (lymphocytes and monocytes) with atypical lymphocytes ('glandular fever cells'). The Paul–Bunnell test (sheep's red-cell agglutination) is positive after the first week or two of illness.

Infectious hepatitis (catarrhal jaundice)

This is the commonest cause of jaundice in children over the age of 3 years. It tends to be milder in children than in adults. There is a prodromal period lasting about a week, in which malaise, anorexia, abdominal pain and nausea predominate, before jaundice appears. (Jaundice is best seen at the periphery of the sclera.) The liver is tender and a little enlarged. The stools are pale, the urine dark, and urine testing reveals the presence of urobilinogen and bile pigment. Urobilinogen may be detected in the pre-icteric stage and may be the sole diagnostic clue in the mildest cases in which clinical jaundice does not develop. Serum bilirubin levels are raised, with roughly equal parts conjugated and free; transaminase levels are raised, and flocculation tests are abnormal.

Differential diagnosis in the pre-icteric and non-icteric cases is from other causes of abdominal pain and vomiting. Once jaundice has developed, diagnosis is not difficult. Complications are very rare. Jaundice usually fades in 1–2 weeks but exceptionally persists for months.

Cross-infection should be prevented as far as possible by care in handling stools and by conscientious hand-washing by the patient and attendants. However, infectivity is greatest before jaundice appears and it is quite common to have more than one case in a household. Diet may be dictated by appetite, which usually means omitting fatty foods and eggs initially. In the average case the child will be confined to bed for a week and kept off school for 2–3 weeks.

TUBERCULOSIS

Tuberculosis is a social indicator disease, being common wherever poverty, malnutrition and overcrowding are prevalent, and rare where standards of hygiene and nutrition are good. In the developing countries of the world tuberculosis appears in forms which were common in Britain 50 years ago. The chief sources of infection are adults with sputum-positive pulmonary tuberculosis, and milk from infected cattle. Prevention depends first upon general improvement in socio-economic conditions, and second upon specific measures including the prompt recognition and treatment of infectious adults, BCG immunization, tuberculin testing of cattle and pasteurization of milk. Mass miniature radiography is of most value where the disease is most prevalent.

The initial infection is in the lungs if conveyed by droplets, in the bowel if conveyed by milk. The first site of infection is known as the primary *focus*: the primary *complex* comprises the primary focus and the enlarged lymph nodes draining it. Spread of infection beyond the local nodes may result in tubercle bacilli reaching the blood stream, causing either tuberculous septicaemia (miliary TB) or infection of distant organs (meninges, kidneys, bones and joints). Tuberculous cervical lymph nodes are thought to be infected via the tonsils. Erythema nodosum may be caused by tuberculosis (p. 210).

In Britain childhood tuberculosis is uncommon. Primary complexes in the lung are seen more often in immigrant children from Asia than in others, and tuberculous meningitis is a rare disease.

Pulmonary tuberculosis

The child with pulmonary TB must not be visualized as an emaciated invalid coughing up blood. Haemoptysis is excessively rare, and systemic symptoms such as fever and weight loss are exceptional. Symptoms are usually minor—malaise, anorexia, cough—and many children with TB traced through their contact with infected adults are completely symptom-free. Diagnosis is based on the X-ray appearances and a positive tuberculin test. Sputum is not usually present, but tubercle bacilli may be recovered from gastric washings. The ESR is usually slightly elevated if the disease is active.

Tuberculous meningitis

This disease which was universally fatal before the discovery of streptomycin is still a serious disease, especially in infancy. It most commonly affects young children and the onset is insidious so that there is usually a history of weight loss or poor weight gain. Initially there is vague malaise, anorexia and perhaps slight fever. After a few days evidence of meningeal involvement is shown by headache, drowsiness, irritability and neck stiffness. If the diagnosis is not made at this stage, convulsions, pareses and impairment of consciousness supervene. The clinical signs are those of meningitis (see p. 91). In addition, choroidal tubercles may be visible as small yellow lesions close to retinal arteries. A careful search must be made with the pupils dilated because the detection of choroidal tubercles is the quickest way of making a certain diagnosis. The CSF may be hazy, and a cobweb clot forms if the fluid is left undisturbed for 24 hours. The cell content is raised, though not extremely so. The cells are predominantly lymphocytes, but polymorphs may predominate in the early stages. Protein is raised: glucose is usually low, but not as low as in pyogenic meningitis. Tubercle bacilli may be seen on suitably stained films of CSF, but their absence does not exclude the diagnosis. Culture and guinea-pig inoculation take several weeks. A chest X-ray may show a localized lesion or miliary lesions. In very sick children the tuberculin test may be negative, and this should never be allowed to exclude the diagnosis. The differential diagnosis is from pyogenic and benign lymphocytic meningitis.

Cervical adenopathy

Tuberculous neck glands are now rare in Britain. Usually a single gland or group of glands is affected, on one side of the neck. The gland is firm (unless caseating), partially fixed and not especially tender. The tuberculin test is positive. The differential diagnosis is from Hodgkin's disease, and infection by anonymous mycobacteria, a group of organisms related to the tubercle bacillus but less virulent. Enlarged glands associated with recurrent tonsillitis are usually bilateral, fairly soft, and mobile, though occasionally they form a localized abscess requiring chemotherapy or drainage.

Management

Regardless of the site the management can be divided into three parts.
1 Notification of the case to the area environmental health specialist so that contacts can be immunized and possible sources of infection identified.
2 Anti-tuberculous drugs. Rifampicin, ethambutol and isoniazid form the basis of treatment in most cases. Treatment should be continued for at least 9 months.
3 General management. Children should not be admitted to hospital or kept off school without good reason. A pulmonary primary complex is rarely infectious, and isolation is often unnecessary. If nutrition is unsatisfactory, it should be improved.

The combination of preventive and therapeutic measures is now so effective that the childhood mortality from tuberculosis has shrunk almost to vanishing point, but only continuing vigilance will keep it this way.

MALARIA

Malaria is endemic in many parts of the world and may be seen in immigrants from malarious areas or in persons who have visited such places but failed to take adequate suppressive drugs. It usually presents with fever which does not necessarily show the classical periodic pattern. The spleen may be enlarged. Diagnosis depends on identification of parasites in blood smears, and may be easier *between* peaks of fever. It may be necessary to examine several smears. Chloroquine is the drug of choice for treatment. For prophylaxis, proguanil (daily) or pyrimethamine (weekly) are used, and must be continued for at least 4 weeks after last exposure.

Further reading

Lawson J. H. *Synospis of Fevers*. Lloyd-Luke, London.

Chapter 22

Accidents and Poisoning

The health of British children is now so good that accidents account for the loss of more lives after the first year of life than does any disease (see p. 298). Road traffic accidents account for nearly half the deaths, and accidents in the home (including burns, falls and poisoning) for about a quarter. Drowning is another important cause of child death. Similarly tragic are the children left with permanent brain damage after severe head injuries and those with extensive scarring from burns and scalds.

Accidents are more common amongst boys than girls. By the age of 11, 1 in 4 children has experienced a serious accident. The risk of accident is influenced by social circumstances. The child in a large family in an industrial slum, on the street much of the day and ostensibly supervised by another child only marginally older, is at great hazard; and the mother trying to care for young children at the top of a tower block, without the privilege of an enclosed garden or play space, has a difficult task. The greatest reduction in mortality and morbidity from accidents will only come about by improved design of towns and homes. Nevertheless, there are many practical things that can be done even in difficult conditions. Injuries to children in car accidents would be reduced to a quarter if all infants were transported in carry cots strapped to the back seat, and if all children wore seat belts in the car. (Any child travelling in a car not fitted with a special child restraint and not large enough to wear an adult belt correctly should be placed in the rear seat with the doors locked to reduce the risk of ejection. On no account should children stand on the car seat because of the risk of being thrown violently forward in an accident). Fireguards, stairgates and locked medicine cupboards are measures that any wise parent should use.

Child-resistant containers for dangerous drugs, and clothes of non-flammable material similarly prevent many accidents. There is great need for better education of children and parents about safety, and for legislation to minimise the opportunities for accidents. Many people feel that it is wrong to enforce the use of protective measures such as seat belts. They feel that individuals should have freedom of choice (regardless of the cost to society or the consequence to others). Children do not have freedom of choice; they cannot choose their parents. They cannot choose parents who will be wise, keeping them in a safe environment. Therefore, legislation is required to minimise the opportunities for accidents to children.

HEAD INJURY

The management of head injuries in children calls for some experience. On the one hand, scalps split easily and bleed profusely, but the quantity of blood may cause unjustifiable alarm. On the other hand, some apparently trivial injuries are associated with intracranial bleeding that only becomes apparent after an interval of time. A history of unconsciousness, however brief, should be regarded seriously. Pallor, vomiting and sleepiness can occur after quite minor injuries, but should settle within an hour or two. Progressive symptoms or the appearance of abnormal neurological signs suggest intracranial injury.

It is customary to have a skull X-ray taken, but a linear fracture without displacement may be unimportant, whilst intracranial bleeding may occur without a fracture. In any case of doubt it is wiser to admit a child with a head injury to hospital for 24 hours' observation, which will include frequent recording of pulse and respiratory rates, blood pressure, level of consciousness and pupillary size and reactions. If there is any suggestion of intracranial bleeding, the opinion of a neurosurgeon should be sought without delay.

BURNS AND SCALDS

Scalds are caused by hot fluids and cause predominantly

loss of the epidermis only, with blistering and peeling. However, the skin of young children sometimes suffers full thickness loss from comparatively minor scalds. For this reason there is a strong argument for limiting the maximum temperature of hot water in the home to 52°C (125°F). Burns are caused by direct contact with very hot objects or by the clothes catching fire and result in full thickness skin loss. The death rate from burns and scalds varies directly with the proportion of the total body surface involved. Loss of skin surface leads to loss of fluid and shock. If more than 10% of the body surface is involved (Fig. 63), intravenous fluid therapy will be

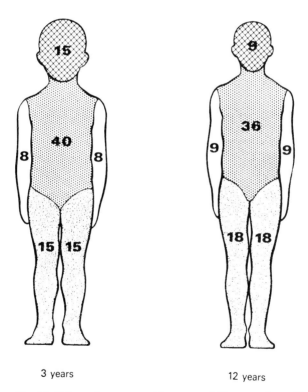

3 years
12 years

Fig. 63. Skin surface areas at 3 years and 12 years of age. The figures indicate the percentage of total body surface represented by each part.

required. Burns involving 50% or more of the body surface carry a grave prognosis, although children have survived much more extensive burns than this. The management of scalds involves the correction of fluid loss, the prevention of infection and the relief of pain. Burns require in addition skin grafting where there has been full thickness skin loss. As a general rule, burns and scalds are more serious than they seem, and hospital admission is advisable for all but the most trivial.

POISONING

The accidental swallowing of drugs and household fluids by young children is extremely common, but remarkably few of them become ill and mortality is very low. The great majority are 2- and 3-year-olds who are sufficiently agile to get hold of things to swallow, but not old enough to appreciate the potential dangers. Occasionally younger children are fed with poisonous substances by their siblings or parents. If older children in the prepubertal–adolescent age range swallow poisonous substances (usually drugs) this is indicative of an emotional upset. Most often it is done as a gesture of defiance, or a wish for temporary oblivion, rather than with serious intention to commit suicide. Nevertheless, some children are pathologically depressed and the advice of a child psychiatrist should be sought when children of this age have swallowed poison.

The things that children swallow are numberless, but fall into three main categories:

1 Tablets and medicines: analgesics, sleeping tablets, tranquillisers, antidepressants and iron are commonly ingested. They are a more common cause of morbidity (and mortality) than substances in the other two groups below.

2 Household and horticultural fluids. Bleach, turpentine, paraffin (kerosene), cleaning fluids and weedkillers form the bulk of this group.

3 Berries and seeds. Laburnum tops the list with deadly nightshade and toadstools featuring commonly. Fortunately, in Britain, things plucked from the hedgerows and ditches hardly ever cause serious illness.

The basis of treatment of poisoning is to minimise

absorption, to promote excretion and to combat symptoms. With some important exceptions, the stomach should be emptied by the most efficient means available unless more than 6 hours have elapsed since the poison was swallowed, or unless it is certain that the amount the child may have swallowed could not cause trouble. For children, most authorities favour induced emesis rather than gastric lavage. It is more effective in removing solid matter (e.g. whole tablets or berries), it is less unpleasant for the child, and it occupies less nursing time. Emesis usually follows the administration of 20 ml ipecacuanha syrup in orange juice, repeated if necessary. Gastric lavage may be needed if emesis does not occur, or if the child is unconscious. The exceptions to the rule of emesis are (a) caustics, such as bleach or acids, which may be presumed from burning around the mouth if there is no adequate history, and (b) hydrocarbons such as turpentine and paraffin. In the case of caustics, the danger of gastric perforation is increased by emesis or lavage: hydrocarbons do little harm in the gastrointestinal tract, but inhalation of vomit may seriously damage the lungs.

Absorption may be discouraged by diluting the poison (milk is good and usually available), by giving an absorbent agent such as activated charcoal, or by giving a specific antidote (e.g. desferrioxamine in iron poisoning). Excretion may be encouraged by the use of purgatives or forced diuresis in selected cases. Supportive treatment in severe cases includes mechanical ventilation for respiratory depression; correction of acid-base balance in aspirin poisoning; and exchange transfusion or peritoneal dialysis in selected cases.

It is usually advisable to admit poisoned children to hospital for observation for at least a few hours. Most major centres now concentrate the management of serious poisoning in specialized units, and a few provide advisory and information services by telephone.

Chronic lead poisoning

Lead poisoning is uncommon in Britain. Lead water pipes have been largely replaced by copper, and drinking water is drawn from main supplies rather than storage tanks. Modern paints for interior decoration contain very little lead, and the British climate does not readily bring to mind the thought of peeling paint on the railings of a sun-baked verandah. Nevertheless, some risks still exist. Amateurs may use lead paints for home decorating or painting cots: lead dust may lie in the vicinity of smelting works or come home on the clothes of lead workers: and disused car batteries are a cheap, if dangerous, form of domestic fuel. Lead may be absorbed by ingestion, inhalation, or through the skin. There may be a history of ingestion of paint or dirt—*pica* (pica is the Latin name for magpie, a bird notorious for stealing and consuming almost anything).

Poisoning is usually chronic and the onset of symptoms is insidious. Early symptoms include abdominal colic, pallor, anaemia, irritability, anorexia and disturbed sleep. Later symptoms are predominantly neurological, including encephalopathy, neuropathy and seizures. Permanent brain damage may result in mental handicap and behaviour disorder. If the onset is more acute, encephalopathic features tend to predominate.

The most difficult part of diagnosis is considering the possibility of lead poisoning. Investigation will then include the measurement of lead levels in blood and urine; estimation of urinary coproporphyrins; X-rays of long bones seeking dense zones at the metaphyses; X-rays of abdomen for opacities within the bowel; and examination of blood films for evidence of hypochromic anaemia and basophil stippling of red cells. Raised lead levels indicate exposure to lead, but not necessarily poisoning.

There is continuing debate and controversy about the significance of marginally elevated blood lead levels, their relationship to abnormal childhood behaviour and the benefit (and cost) that might accrue from reducing the lead content of petrol.

NON-ACCIDENTAL INJURY ('battered babies')

It may seem inappropriate to discuss deliberate injury to children in a chapter on accidents, but in spite of much publicity about battered babies doctors still fail to recognize the true nature of some childhood injuries. Although children of any age may be physically abused, babies under 6 months are especially vulnerable. The true incidence is unknown but is certainly not less than 5 per 1000 children.

There are probably 4000 children in Britain who are injured through purposeful acts of their parents each year, and of these about 400 die. At least an equal number suffer permanent injury leading to mental impairment or neurological abnormality (cerebral palsy).

No parents are immune to the possibility of striking their child in anger, but certain features commonly underlie child abuse.

The parents have often been subject to cruelty in their own childhood. The injured child cries excessively and is overdemanding. The home is overcrowded so that parents and children are constantly on top of one another. Father may be on shift-work and attempting to sleep when the family is awake.

Injury and neglect are closely associated and are both indications of parental inadequacy. The child with non-accidental injury may, therefore, also show evidence of poor standards of hygiene or nutrition, although most are well-fed. The family may already be known to the health visitor as in need of supervision. In other cases one child is singled out for abuse whilst the rest of the family appear well cared for. The most common forms of deliberate injury are shown in Fig. 64. They are:

1   Bruising, especially of the face and trunk. The bruises may be multiple and of different ages. (It is important to realise that a normal active toddler is likely to have five or six bruises of different ages on him.)

2   Fractures, especially of the ribs, humerus and femur. Such fractures in infancy should always alert the doctor.

3   Head injury. Skull fracture and subdural haematoma may occur together or separately. Retinal and sub-hya-loid haemorrhages are a common accompaniment. The most severe head injuries will cause intraventricular and intracerebral haemorrhage leading to death or per-manent brain damage.

4   Burns, either from cigarettes or from holding the child close to a fire.

The doctor's suspicions should be aroused by the history if (a) there has been an inexplicable delay in seeking medical advice, which may even be as long as a

few days; (b) the explanation given for the injuries is not

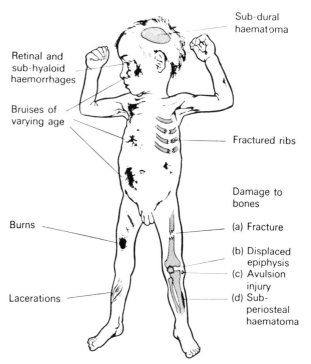

Retinal and
sub-hyaloid
haemorrhages

Bruises of
varying age

Burns

Lacerations

Sub-dural
haematoma

Fractured ribs

Damage to
bones

(a) Fracture

(b) Displaced
epiphysis
(c) Avulsion
injury
(d) Sub-
periosteal
haematoma

Fig. 64. Injuries sustained by battered babies.

compatible with their severity. For example, a baby's skull does not fracture if he rolls off the sofa on to a carpeted floor. If there is any reasonable suspicion of deliberate injury the child must be admitted to hospital for his own safety. A careful clinical record of bruises and other skin lesions must be made, with drawings and photographs. A skeletal X-ray survey may show unsuspected fractures at various stages of healing.

The doctor's function is not to act as detective or judge, even less as public prosecutor, but to safeguard his patient and help the family. The NSPCC and social services department may well be enlisted to help, and in some areas the police adopt a constructive attitude. Social services departments maintain registers of children who have incurred physical injury or neglect,

282

failure to thrive and emotional abuse, with the purpose of preventing neglect or damage to other children in those households. Court action may be necessary to take a child into the care of the local authority if the risk of further assault is felt to be substantial. Further abuse occurs in up to 20% of cases, but the recurrence rate is a sensitive index of the effectiveness of management. If there is skilled, intensive, continuous help for these families, recurrence can be altogether avoided.

COT DEATH (sudden unexplained death of infancy)

The sudden death of an infant which is unexpected by history, and in which a thorough post-mortem examination fails to demonstrate an adequate cause, occurs in just under 3 per 1000 live births. In the United Kingdom cot deaths constitute about one-fifth of infant deaths.

Most occur at home between the ages of 4 weeks and 4 months, in urban rather than rural areas, during the night, and in late winter and early spring, when community respiratory infections are most prevalent. They are frequently preceded by symptoms of minor illness, they are more common in males, in twins, in infants of low birth weight, and in the socially and economically deprived. The infant's mothers tend to be younger and to have had more children when compared to controls. They do not keep antenatal clinic appointments for themselves or follow-up clinic appointments for the babies.

On closer enquiry, some infants found dead in their cots have shown signs of ill health for at least a few hours beforehand, and post-mortem examination, if sufficiently detailed, reveals an explanation. Most of these children have unsatisfactory social backgrounds. Other infants have been perfectly well prior to death and no explanation is found at autopsy. They come from all social classes. Many hypotheses have been proposed to explain these unexplained cot deaths but substantial proof has been lacking. In recent years evidence has accumulated suggesting that abnormalities of the ventilatory control mechanism may be important. Babies with mild upper airways infection tend to develop periodic respiration with attacks of apnoea (rather like that seen in pre-term babies). It seems that viraemia may upset the respiratory control mechanism and that some sudden infant deaths may be the result of unduly prolonged apnoea.

Further reading

Apley J., Mac Keith R. C. and Meadow S. R. The Environment, the Family and the Child. Chapter 3, *The Child and his Symptoms*. Blackwell Scientific Publications.

Black J. A. *Paediatric Emergencies*, Butterworths.

Jackson R. H. *Children, The Environment and Accidents*, Pitman Medical.

Franklin A. W. *Concerning Child Abuse*. Churchill Livingstone.

Chapter 23

Children in Society

The health and educational progress of a child is directly related to the home and the environment. The child of an unskilled worker (social class V) has a 50% greater chance of being born dead or with a serious physical handicap than a lawyer's child (social class I). The disadvantage is there at birth and continues throughout childhood. The social class IV or V child will have more accidents, more physical illnesses, will be smaller and will read less well than the child from social class I or II. The Registrar-General's five-point grading of social class is a crude but useful classification. Although it depends on the occupation of the father, we recognize that the father's occupation has close correlation with many other important factors including income, housing and attitudes to child rearing. In Britain the proportion of families in each social class is approximately:

I	Higher professional (usually university graduates)	5%
II	Other professional and technical	15%
III	Other non-manual and skilled manual	55%
IV	Semi-skilled manual	19%
V	Unskilled manual	6%

Family size and birth order can also be important, particularly for 5th and subsequent children who tend to be smaller and have an increased chance of death in infancy or handicap later on.

Despite the liberalisation of the abortion laws, the proportion of children born out of wedlock (i.e. illegitimate) has risen to 12% of all live births. A third of them are born to young women under 20, and most stay with their mother or grandparents in what is often an unsatisfactory home. The change in the traditional pattern of family life, and the increase in marriage breakdown has resulted in more than 1/8th of all families with children being single-parent families.

Unsatisfactory homes are not just those where there is overt cruelty, poverty or squalor. Stress at home may result from parental discord—quarrelling and separations, one parent families, and children who have been put in the care of the wrong parent after divorce. It may result from parental illness—a dying or chronically handicapped mother, a mentally ill father—or just from parental inadequacy—work-shy parents, drunken parents and those who have given up the struggle of trying to be satisfactory parents.

The doctor sees the childhood casualties of these situations: poor development, illness and behavioural problems, or children who have to stay in hospital because of the home situation rather than the severity of the illness. The teacher sees the casualties also; unhappy children, delinquent children and children with school problems.

The complexity and multiplicity of factors that cause a child to be disadvantaged sometimes fills the doctor or other helper with a feeling of hopelessness. However, since bad factors multiply each other's effect, conversely great benefit may be achieved by modifying even one bad factor. Even when everything seems hopeless it is worth trying to modify one or two definite fields of the child's life to try to achieve for that child at least one of the following:
1   Self-esteem
2   One good relationship with another person
3   Firm supervision and discipline.

Elaborate local authority medical and social services exist particularly for disadvantaged children. But all too often the services are best used by the child of well-informed middle-class parents, while the socially disadvantaged child cannot use them, because his parents either do not know or do not care. Therefore all medical and para-medical staff have a constant duty to detect children in need or in distress and to see that they have the opportunity to benefit from the help that is available.

Some of the more important services are summarized in this chapter. (See also Appendix 6, p. 307.)

COMMUNITY MEDICAL SERVICES

Health visitors

These are registered nurses who also hold a midwifery qualification and a health visitor's certificate. They are employed by the health authority though an increasing number are being allocated to group general practices and a few have hospital attachments. They are responsible for family health, and particularly that of mothers and children. Their job is to prevent illness and handicap by the early detection of problems and mobilisation of services to deal with those problems. Their duties range from screening 9-month-old infants for deafness and advising mothers of young children, to being the friend and helper of old folk who live alone. They have an important role in health education.

Child health clinics (infant welfare clinics)

These are organised by the health authority and are staffed by health visitors and ancillary workers. Most of the doctors who work at these centres do so on a part-time sessional basis and may be general practitioners. Their role is a supervisory one; they aim to provide routine medical examination of infants and pre-school children and to ensure optimal physical, emotional and mental development for the child. They provide immunization services and health education for new mothers, as well as advising and supporting those who have problems. Ninety per cent of babies attend such a clinic at least once in the first year, but after the age of 2 attendance drops sharply.

EDUCATION AND THE SCHOOL HEALTH SERVICE

The school health service was established in 1904 to investigate the reason why 40% of young people volunteering for service in the Boer war were found to be medically unfit. Today its main function is to assess the state of health of schoolchildren, help with the problems created by ill-health, and to promote better health. The service is particularly important for children from unsatisfactory homes who may have missed the voluntary pre-school health checks.

The service is separated off to some extent from other medical services so that those in the service can work in close collaboration with the education department and local paediatricians.

School medical officers, many of whom are part-time workers, are responsible for identifying schoolchildren with disorders which are likely to interfere with their development, education and happiness. The traditional annual 5-minute inspection of every child is being replaced by more detailed assessment of a few selected children about whom the teachers are worried.

In some towns the school health service still provides 'school clinics', held in educational premises and organised like a children's outpatient clinic or therapy session, e.g. ENT, orthopaedic and dental clinics, and physiotherapy, speech therapy and orthoptic services. The trend is for these school clinics to be transferred to health service premises.

Special School facilities are provided by the education department for children requiring special education. There are schools for:

Educationally subnormal (moderate)—ESN(M)

Educationally subnormal (severe)—ESN(S)

Physically handicapped (e.g. cerebral palsy or spina bifida)

Hearing impairment—(a) deaf (b) partially hearing

Visual impairment—(a) blind (b) partially sighted

Epileptic

Maladjusted (psychological disorders)

Communication problems (other than the deaf)

Delicate (a small and decreasing number of children who do not fit into the other categories, but cannot manage at normal school because of e.g. intractable asthma. They are used mainly for educational and psychological convalescence.)

No child is sent to a special school who can be educated satisfactorily in an ordinary school. Though only 1·5% of children will be in a special school at any one time, 15% of children receive special education for some period of their school days.

Most areas will have adequate facilities for children who are ESN or physically handicapped—the disorders are common. But for less common disorders the child may have to be a boarder far from home and the local authority pays. For instance, there are at present only two schools of 'grammar school' level for blind children in England.

The special schools play an important role in the welfare of handicapped children; but most parents want their child to attend a normal school if at all possible. The extra staff and facilities of the special school are outweighed in their minds by the inconvenience, the social stigma of being different, and the lower academic standard of most special schools. Therefore, increased integration is the modern aim with handicapped children attending ordinary schools, and the provision of special classes for handicapped children in larger schools.

Nursery schools

These exist as separate schools or as nursery classes attached to primary schools. They cater for children aged 3–5 and are run by specially trained teachers assisted by nursery assistants and nurses. They aim to encourage a child's development and learning by play, stimulation and physical activity.

There is a great shortage of these schools and classes, and at present under 5% of children can be accommodated; the number who would benefit is many times that proportion. Priority is given to children with social or medical handicap, and to those with mothers who go out to work.

DEPARTMENT OF SOCIAL SERVICES

The social services department is responsible for the care and/or supervision of children up to 18 years in a variety of circumstances. A child may be accommodated by the local authority if he cannot be cared for by his parents or guardians temporarily or permanently, by reason of their illness or death, or because the child has been abandoned or lost. In certain circumstances the local authority may be designated a 'fit person' to assume parental rights in order to provide security and protection for the child.

Parental rights may be given to the local authority by the Court (usually the Juvenile Court) in which case, a child is said to be the subject of a *care order*. In Britain over 90,000 children are in care. Grounds for a care order include health impairment, neglect of proper development, ill treatment, moral danger, failure to attend school, incitement to crime, or being beyond the control of parent or guardian. The child has to be in need of care and control which is unlikely to be received unless a care order is made. The local authority tries to keep or place children with their own parents, relatives or friends whether care is temporary, permanent, voluntary or through a court order. When this is not possible local authority accommodation is used. It includes:

1 *Foster homes* in which a child is cared for in a family other than his own. Half the children 'in care' are in foster homes; brief placements are successful, but long-term fostering tends to be unsuccessful. There are an increasing number of schemes in which the foster parents are paid additional money to look after children with physical and mental handicap or disturbed adolescents.

2 *Children's homes* are usually run on 'family' lines, aiming to provide as normal an upbringing as possible, despite frequent changes of staff. They contain a higher proportion of difficult or handicapped children than foster homes. Ninety-five percent of children in these homes still have a living parent, so that many are visited regularly or may be reunited with their parents for weekends or longer periods in the future. Children's homes are much more expensive for the local authority than fostering.

3 *Hostels for working children*

4 *Residential nurseries*

5 *Community homes* (formerly approved schools): Children may now be placed directly into these homes.

Children are also supervised in their own homes either on a voluntary basis or as a result of a court *supervision order*: the social worker's prime aim here is to prevent family break-up and to try to help with problems of care, physical and emotional. The social worker is always glad to work as part of a team with others involved with the family, e.g. health visitors, doctors, teachers.

The social services department is also responsible for

supervising children placed privately with foster parents. People who look after other people's children, whether on a day (child day-care, childminder) or residential (foster) basis, must register with their local social services department, even though they may be paid direct by the parent.

Day nurseries

These are for pre-school children and cater for two main groups of children (1) those who require day-time care whilst their parents are at work or ill—particularly those who only have a single parent. (2) Children from poor quality homes where stimulation and company are lacking. The number of day nurseries is few and the demand large. This has led to groups of parents forming their own centres for pre-school children, variously named *play groups*, play centres, crèches, etc. Most of these groups require considerable parent participation and organization and at present are mainly run by middle-class parents for their middle-class children.

VOLUNTARY SERVICES

The statutory services are supplemented by a large number of voluntary and charitable organizations. Some of these organizations were amongst the first to provide any help for disadvantaged children. The NSPCC (National Society for the Prevention of Cruelty to Children) continues its historic role of providing support and advice for families under stress. Barnardo's continues to provide good happy residential care for homeless and handicapped children. Other organizations are relatively new. The Spastics Society provides medical and educational services for children with cerebral palsy in addition to sponsoring a large research programme.

ADOPTION

Couples wishing to adopt a baby should approach either their local authority or a registered adoption society. Each agency tends to have its own requirements, for instance attachment to a particular religious denomination or an age limit—it is difficult to adopt a child if you are over 40. The agencies' main concern will be relationships within the family, but it is also important for applicants to have a steady income, a settled home and satisfactory health. Once accepted the applicants have to wait anything from a few months to 3 years, until a suitable baby is placed with them. A child of any age under 18 may be adopted but the most usual placements are of illegitimate babies. The natural mother, and in some circumstances the father, is asked to sign a form agreeing to the adoption. There is a minimum 3 months' probationary period, during which the natural mother can claim the baby back; about 2% do. During this period the applicants will be visited by a social worker as will all the people concerned in the adoption. At the end of this time, if parental consents are signed and confirmed and reports on the adoptive home are satisfactory, the adoption order will be made in court. The child is now a full member of the adoptive family; he takes their name and has all the rights of a natural child (except that he cannot inherit a title!).

Medical examinations are required for both parents, for the baby before placement and again before the adoption hearing. It is essential to explain and discuss any suspected handicaps with the prospective parents. Parents are also advised to inform their child from the beginning that they are adopted and to explain this regularly and more fully as the child's understanding increases.

The increased tolerance shown by society to unmarried mothers, and the increased financial and practical support available for them have resulted in fewer babies being offered for adoption. There is now a shortage of healthy non-coloured babies for adoption, and an excess of childless couples wishing to adopt.

Pregnant women seeking advice about adoption should be advised to approach their social services department or a recognised voluntary organisation specialising in helping the unmarried mother.

A leaflet for prospective adopters which gives the necessary details about adoption societies is available from the British Adoption and Fostering Agencies, 4 Southampton Row, London WC1B 4AA.

LAWS RELATING TO THE YOUNG

For legal purposes a child remains a 'child' up to the age of 14, is a 'young person' up to 17, and is an adult at 18. However, many laws become operative at other ages.

School

School education is compulsory for children aged 5 and over. Children may not leave until they are 16.

Work

Children may not be employed until they are 13. Then they may be employed only between the hours of 7 am and 7 pm, and for a maximum of 2 hours on school days.

Abuse

It is an offence to:
tattoo anyone under 18,
seduce a girl under 16,
sell tobacco to a child under 16,
sell fireworks to a child under 13,
expose to fire risk (e.g. not use a fire guard) a child under 12,
give intoxicating liquor to children under 5.

Crime

Children under 10 (under 8 in Scotland) are not considered 'criminally responsible' for their misdeeds, and may be dealt with by Juvenile Courts.

The Court can make (1) a 'Care Order' giving parental rights to the local authority or (2) a 'Supervision Order' which may be administered by the social services department or, if the child is over 14, by the probation department. At the age of 15 children can be sent to Borstal.

Adult courts deal with those over the age of 17. Although it is legally possible to be sent to prison for a first offence at the age of 17, it is in practice rare before the age of 20.

At the age of 100 the child receives a telegram of congratulation from the Queen.

Chapter 24

Mortality and Morbidity

The health of nations has traditionally been measured by mortality. It seems paradoxical, but it is administratively relatively easy to ensure the notification of deaths and their causes to health authorities. Morbidity is more difficult to determine except for a few diseases, mostly infections, which are notifiable by law. Special studies are needed to determine the prevalence of other conditions.

The causes of death and patterns of illness in children are markedly different from those in adults. They are influenced by a diversity of factors which include sex, legitimacy, social class, place of birth and season. The secular decline in child mortality during the present century has resulted more from preventive measures than from improved treatment.

Child mortality is concentrated in the perinatal period, and the only remaining scope for a *major* reduction in child deaths lies in better obstetric, neonatal and infant care.

Important mortality indices include:

Stillbirth rate	=	Stillbirths per 1000 total births
Perinatal mortality rate	=	Stillbirths + first week deaths per 1000 total births
Neonatal mortality rate	=	Deaths in first 28 days per 1000 live births
Infant mortality rate	=	Deaths in first year per 1000 live births

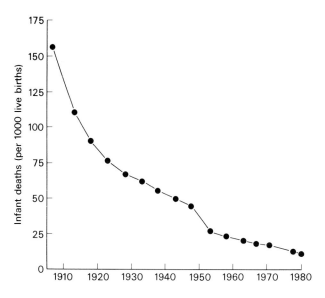

Fig. 65. Infant Mortality (0–1 year). By 1979 the infant mortality rate in England and Wales had fallen to one twelfth of the level in 1900—from 156 to 12·8 per 1000 live births. The present rate is amongst the lowest in the world but by no means the lowest in Europe (see Table 17).

Table 17. Infant mortality rates (IMR): International League Table 1977

1st Division (I.M.R. < 10)		3rd Division (I.M.R. 15–19)	
Sweden	8·0	Belgium	15·3*
Denmark	8·7	W. Germany	15·5
Japan	8·9	Spain	15·6
		Eire	15·7
2nd Division (I.M.R. 10–14)		Scotland	16·1
Norway	9·1	Austria	16·8
Iceland	9·5	N. Ireland	17·2
Netherlands	9·5	Italy	17·7
Switzerland	9·8	Israel	17·8
France	11·5	Czechoslovakia	19·6
Finland	12·0		
Canada	12·4	**4th Division (I.M.R. 20–24)**	
Australia	12·5	Greece	20·3
E. Germany	13·1	Poland	24·6
England and Wales	13·8		
U.S.A.	14·0	**Also ran**	
New Zealand	14·2	Hungary	26·6
		U.S.S.R.	27·7†
		Romania	31·2
		Yugoslavia	35·2

* 1976 figure.
† 1974 figure, excluding first week deaths of very small infants.

Table 18. Episodes of childhood illness in general practice in one year 1975/76

Diagnosis	Episodes per 1000 children	
	0–4 years	5–14 years
All causes	2824	1371
Upper respiratory infections; cough	900	398
Otitis media	198	82
Lower respiratory infections	142	61
Enteritis; diarrhoea; vomiting	144	36
Specific infectious diseases	79	49
Conjunctivitis	87	26
Skin infections	38	41
Urinary infections	10	6
Unexplained fever	24	6
Rash	43	12
Dermatitis and eczema	116	28
Urticaria	12	10
Trauma	67	91
Asthma	9	12
Behavioural disorders	30	10
Insomnia	10	1
Constipation	13	6
Enuresis	5	9

Pre-school children are seen by their GP on average three times a year, school-age children once or twice. Infections, especially of the upper respiratory tract, account for more episodes of illness than all other causes together. Data from Royal College of General Practitioners.

Table 19. Social class and childhood mortality, England and Wales, 1970–72. Death rates per 100,000

	Social class				
	I	II	III	IV	V
All causes (age)					
1–4 years	59	58	69	89	119
5–9 years	27	28	35	38	57
10–14 years	25	26	28	33	45
Age 1–4 years					
Accidents, poisoning, violence	9	14	17	25	45
Respiratory disease	13	9	13	17	21
Neoplasms	9	9	9	9	12
Congenital abnormalities	12	12	12	15	13
Asthma	1	1	0·5	0·5	0·5

At any age a child from social class V is twice as likely to die as one from social class I. The most conspicuous rise in death rate is between classes IV and V. At ages 1–4 years there is little social class difference in deaths from neoplasms and congenital abnormalities, and for asthma the general trend is reversed.

Table 20. Deaths of children by age group, England and Wales, 1979, all causes

	Age						
	1st day	Remainder of 1st week	Remainder of 1st month	Remainder of 1st year	1–4 years	5–9 years	10–14 years
Males	1381	1168	538	1644	641	602	605
Females	983	775	411	1278	527	368	386
Total	2364	1943	949	2922	1168	970	991
M/F ratio	1·40	1·51	1·31	1·29	1·22	1·64	1·57

It is apparent that childhood deaths are concentrated early in life, and that death rates at all ages in childhood are appreciably higher for boys than for girls.

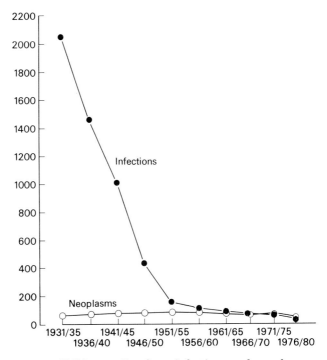

Fig. 66. Child mortality from infections and neoplasms, 1931–1980. There has been a dramatic decline in child deaths from infections, from over 2000 to 15 per million children living, aged 1–14 years. The decline was as dramatic before the introduction of sulphonamides and antibiotics as subsequently. Over the same period, death rates from neoplasm have not changed significantly.

INCIDENCE OF SOME IMPORTANT PROBLEMS

10% of 1-year-old boys have been circumcised.

7% of 5-year-olds have had at least one convulsion.
5% of 5-year-olds have a squint.
5% of 5-year-olds have a behavioural problem.
5% of 5-year-olds have a speech or language problem.
2% of 5-year-olds have a substantial congenital defect.

16% of 7-year-olds have had tonsillectomy or adenoidectomy.
2% of 7-year-olds have had a hernia repair.
1% of 7-year-olds have had an appendicectomy.
10% of 7-year-olds wet their beds.
10% of 7-year-olds have eczema, asthma or hay fever.
13% of 7-year-olds require special education.
5% of 7-year-olds receive special education.

INCIDENCE OF SOME NOTORIOUS CONDITIONS

Many conditions about which you have learnt, and some of which you will have seen in large regional children's centres, are very rare. Professor Illingworth of Sheffield has calculated the average length of time that a British general practitioner (with a practice of 2500 patients) would have to work to see a child presenting with one of the following conditions:

	Years
Pyloric stenosis	4
Mental subnormality	4
Congenital heart disease	5
Spina bifida	6
Diabetes mellitus	6
Epilepsy	6
Cot death	8
Intussusception	12
Hydrocephalus	12
Mongol	16
Congenital dislocation of the hip	37
Turner's syndrome	60
Oesophageal atresia	75

	Years
Autism	120
Adrenogenital syndrome	200
Phenylketonuria	240
Cretinism	250
Malignant disease	250
Nephrotic syndrome	350
Muscular dystrophy	480
Haemophilia	600
Hirschsprung's disease	600
Galactosaemia	1725
Tay–Sachs disease	6250

Appendixes

Appendix I. Head circumference chart

Appendix 2. Weight and height centile table for boys

Age	Weight (kg)			Height (cm)		
	3%	50%	97%	3%	50%	97%
Birth	2·5	3·5	4·4		50	
3 months	4·4	5·7	7·2	55	60	64
6 ,,	6·2	7·8	9·8	62	66·5	71
9 ,,	7·6	9·3	11·6	66·5	71	76
12 ,,	8·4	10·3	12·8	70	75	80
15 ,,	9·0	11	13·6	73	78	84
18 ,,	9·4	11·7	14·2	75	81	87
21 ,,	9·8	12·2	14·9	78	84	90
2 years	10·2	12·7	16	80	87	93
2½ ,,	10·9	13·7	17	84	92	99
3 ,,	11·6	14·7	18	86	95	103
3½ ,,	12·5	15·8	19	90	98	106
4 ,,	13	17	20	94	101	110
4½ ,,	14	18	22	96	105	114
5 ,,	14·5	19	23	100	108	117
6 ,,	16	21	25	105	114	124
7 ,,	17	23	28	110	120	130
8 ,,	19	25	31	115	126	137
9 ,,	21	27	35	120	132	143
10 ,,	23	30	39	125	137	148
11 ,,	25	34	43	128	142	154
12 ,,	27	38	49	133	147	160
13 ,,	30	43	55	137	151	165
14 ,,	33	48	62	142	157	172
15 ,,	39	55	67	148	163	179

Head circumference (cm) for boys

	3%	50%	97%
Birth	33	35	38
12 months	45	47	49
18 ,,	46	49	51
2 years	47	50	52
3 ,,	48	50	53
5 ,,	49	51	54
8 ,,	50	52	55
12 ,,	51	54	56
14 ,,	53	56	58

Appendix 3. Weight and height centile table for girls

Age	Weight (kg)			Height (cm)		
	3%	50%	97%	3%	50%	97%
Birth	2·5	3·5	4·4		50	
3 months	4·4	5·6	7·2	55	60	65
6 ,,	6·2	7·8	9·3	62	67	72
9 ,,	7·8	9·2	11·6	65	71	76
12 ,,	8·4	10·3	12·8	70	75	80
15 ,,	9·0	11·0	13·6	73	78	84
18 ,,	9·4	11·6	14·2	75	81	87
21 ,,	9·8	12·2	14·8	78	84	90
2 years	10·2	12·7	15·5	80	87	93
2½ ,,	11	13·7	16·7	84	92	99
3 ,,	11·6	14·7	18	85	95	104
3½ ,,	12	15	19	90	97	105
4 ,,	13	16	20	93	100	108
4½ ,,	14	17	21	96	104	112
5 ,,	15	18	22	99	107	116
6 ,,	16	19	25	104	114	123
7 ,,	18	22	28	109	120	129
8 ,,	19	24	32	114	125	135
9 ,,	21	26	36	118	130	142
10 ,,	23	29	41	123	135	148
11 ,,	25	33	46	128	141	156
12 ,,	28	37	52	133	147	161
13 ,,	31	41	57	139	153	167
14 ,,	36	46	62	145	158	170
15 ,,	40	51	67	149	160	172

Head circumference (cm) for girls

	3%	50%	97%
Birth	33	35	38
12 months	43	46	48
18 ,,	45	47	50
2 years	46	48	51
3 ,,	47	49	52
5 ,,	48	50	53
8 ,,	50	52	54
12 ,,	51	53	56
14 ,,	52	54	57

Appendix 4. Teeth

There are 20 deciduous and 32 permanent teeth

Deciduous		Appearance
Central Incisor	lower	6–10 months
	upper	7–10 ,,
Lateral Incisor	upper	8–10 ,,
	lower	12–18 ,,
First Molar		12–18 ,,
Canine		16–20 ,,
Second Molar		20–30 ,,

Permanent teeth appear from the 6th year. The first molars and central incisors appear first. All teeth have appeared by the age of 14 except the third molars. Teeth appear a few months earlier in girls.

A fluoride content of 1 part per million in the water results in 30–50% less caries. Therefore, in the many areas in which fluoride content is low, a fluoride supplement is advisable, particularly during the first 8 years of life.

Appendix 5. Measurement and conversion

To Metric

One ounce	= 28·4 grams (g)
One pound	= 0·45 kilogram (kg)
One fluid ounce	= 28·4 millilitres (ml)
One pint	= 0·56 litre (l)*
One inch	= 2·54 centimetre (cm)

From Metric

One kilogram	= 2·2 pounds (lb)
One litre	= 1·76 pints
One centimetre	= 0·39 inch (in.)

* The United States' pint contains 16 fluid ounces, i.e. 0·45 litre.

Appendix 6. A programme of child health surveillance

(adapted from *Prevention in the Child Health Services*, published by DHSS, 1980)

Every effort should be made to ensure that women of child-bearing age are themselves healthy and that, by sensible family planning, pregnancies are welcome.

I Monitoring development

1 *Programme Schedule*

   (a) At birth. Clinical examination (see p. 14) (doctor or midwife).
   (b) At 6–10 days. Full clinical examination (doctor).
   (c) 6 weeks. Assessment of well-being, weight gain and development (health visitor).
   (d) 7–8 months. Review of development. Screening tests for vision and hearing (health visitor with medical back-up).
   (e) 18 months. Review of development, especially social and language (health visitor). Opportunity to discuss toilet training.
   (f) About 3 years. General review including hearing, vision, squint, teeth. Opportunity to discuss emotional and social problems.
   (g) School entry. Comprehensive medical examination during first school year.
   (h) School years. Regular checks of growth, hearing, vision, teeth. Testing of colour vision (especially boys) at 8–9 years. Examination of children about whom parents or teachers are concerned. Opportunities for older children to refer themselves to school doctor or nurse.

2 *Screening tests*
   (a) Hearing and vision as above.
   (b) Congenital dislocation of the hip—at birth, 6–10 days, 6 weeks.
   (c) Phenylketonuria and hypothyroidism at 4–8 days.

II Immunization

   See page 263.

III Health education and preparation for parenthood

During the final years at school and further education, and in the antenatal period, there are numerous opportunities for health education. As a contribution towards reducing child mortality and morbidity, the following matters deserve emphasis:

   (i) the dangers of delaying antenatal care,

  (ii) the importance of good nutrition,

 (iii) the adverse effects of smoking and of immoderate drinking during pregnancy upon the unborn baby,

 (iv) the importance of fondling and talking to babies and of play,

  (v) the importance of breast feeding: the proper techniques of bottle feeding if the baby is not breast fed,

 (vi) the relationship between parental smoking and respiratory disease in children,

(vii) how to recognise when a child is ill,

(viii) how to minimise the risks of accidents at home and on the road,

 (ix) the importance of dental health,

  (x) the role of the father.

Appendix 7. Developmental milestones*

Posture and movement	*Vision and manipulation*
3 months	
Prone: rests on forearms, lifts up head and chest.	Vision: alert, watches movement of adult.
Pulled to sit: head bobs forward, then held erect.	Follows dangling toy held 6 inches from face.
Held standing: sags at knees	Hands: loosely open.
6 months	
Prone: lifts up on extended arms. Pulls self to sit, and sits erect with support.	Watches rolling ball 2 yards away. Reaches out for toy and takes in palmar grasp, puts to mouth.
Held standing: takes weight on legs.	
9 months	
Prone: wriggles or crawls.	Looks for toys that are dropped.
Sits unsupported for 10 minutes.	Scissor grasp and transfer to other hand before placing object in mouth.
Held standing: bounces or stamps.	
1 year	
Crawls on all fours.	Drops toys deliberately and watches where they go.
Walks round furniture stepping side-ways. Walks with hands held.	Index finger approach to tiny objects, then pincer grasp.
Stands alone for a second or two.	
1½ years	
Walks alone and can pick up a toy from floor without falling.	Builds tower of three cubes. Scribbles.
2 years	
Runs.	Builds tower of six cubes.
Walks up and down stairs two feet to a step.	
3 years	
Walks upstairs one foot per step, and down two feet per step.	Builds tower of nine cubes. Copies a ○.
Stands on one foot momentarily.	
4 years	
Walks up and down stairs one foot per step.	Builds three steps from six cubes (after demonstration).
Stands on one foot for 5 seconds.	Copies a ○ and ×.
5 years	
Skips. Hops.	Draws a man.
Stands on one foot with arms folded for 5 seconds.	Copies ○, × and □.

* Average age of achievements

Hearing and speech	*Social behaviour*
Quietens to interesting sounds. Chuckles and coos when pleased.	Shows pleasure appropriately.
Localizes soft sounds 18 inches lateral to either ear. Makes double syllable sounds and tuneful noises.	Alert, interested. Still friendly with strangers.
Brisk localisation of soft sounds 3 feet lateral to either ear. Babbles tunefully.	Distinguishes strangers and shows apprehension. Chews solids.
Understands simple commands. Babbles incessantly.	Cooperates with dressing, e.g. holding up arms. Waves bye-bye.
Uses several words, sound labels.	Drinks from cup using two hands. Demands constant mothering.
Joins words together in simple phrases, as sound ideas.	Uses spoon. Indicates toilet needs, dry by day.
Speaks in sentences. Gives full name.	Eats with spoon and fork. Can undress with assistance. Dry by night.
Talks a lot. Speech contains many infantile substitutions.	Dresses and undresses with assistance.
Fluent speech with few infantile substitutions.	Dresses and undresses alone. Washes and dries face and hands.

Appendix 8. Further reading

At the end of most chapters we have listed one or two books for further reading or reference. In addition there are many comprehensive paediatric text books and specialist monographs—more than enough to suit all tastes. Those which we find particularly useful and which are likely to be in the local library are:

Large comprehensive textbooks

Forfar J. O. and Arneil G. C. *Textbook of Paediatrics*, Churchill-Livingstone.
Vaughan V. C. and McKay R. J. *Nelson's Textbook of Paediatrics*. W. B. Saunders.

Medium-sized books

Hutchinson J. H. *Practical Paediatric Problems*. Lloyd Luke.
Jolly H. *Diseases of Children*, Blackwell Scientific Publications.
Mitchell R. *Child Health in the Community*. Churchill-Livingstone.
Nixon H. H. and O'Donnell B. *The Essentials of Paediatric Surgery*. Heinemann.

Other books

Clinics in Developmental Medicine is a series of monographs on neurological and developmental aspects of children, published by Heinemann.
Scientific Foundations of Paediatrics. Edited by Davis J. A. and Dobbing J. Heinemann. This comprehensive reference book contains detailed information about the scientific background to growth and development.
Clinical Paediatric Physiology. Edited by Godfrey S. and Baum J. D., Blackwell Scientific Publications.
Paediatric Chemical Pathology. Clinical Tests and Reference Ranges. Clayton B. E., Jenkins P., J. M., Blackwell Scientific Publications.

Reviews

Topical reviews on selected subjects are available in the following periodic publications:
Advances in Paediatrics. Year Book Medical Publishers.
Recent Advances in Paediatrics. Churchill.
The Paediatric Clinics of North America. W. B. Saunders.

Books for parents

Jolly H. *The Book of Child Care*. Sphere.
Spock B. *Baby and Child Care*

Index